To my dear husband and best friend, Dan.
Your unfailing support has given me the courage
to dream, to challenge, and, finally, to write.

DAWN GROVES

YOGA

FOR BUSY PEOPLE

INCREASE ENERGY
AND REDUCE STRESS
IN MINUTES A DAY

NEW WORLD LIBRARY
Novato, California

New World Library
14 Pamaron Way, Novato, CA 94949

© 1995 Dawn Groves

Cover design: Greg Wittrock
Text design: TBH Typecast, Inc.
Typesetting: Stephanie Eichleay
Editorial: Gina Misiroglu
Illustrations: Marilynn Grant Barr

Library of Congress Cataloging-in-Publication Data

Groves, Dawn, 1955–
Yoga for busy people : increase energy and reduce stress in
minutes a day / Dawn Groves.
p.   cm.
Includes bibliographical references.
ISBN 1-880032-47-3 : $10.95
1. Yoga, Hatha.   I. Title.
RA781.7G76   1995   94-40501
613.7'046--dc20   CIP

First Printing, February, 1995
ISBN 1-880032-47-3
Printed in Canada on acid-free paper
Distributed by Publishers Group West
10 9 8

Acknowledgments

A completed book is a compendium of interest and effort from a number of important contributors. Thank you Alamaia, my first yoga teacher, not only for offering your vast knowledge, but for instilling in me a deep respect and love for yoga. Heartfelt thanks go to the sensitive, skilled yoga instructors who unselfishly reviewed and commented on the postures and techniques described in this text. Specifically, thank you Joan Bauer for your generous commentary and thoughtful support. Thank you Dr. Marilyn Hall-Day, founding minister at the New Thought Center for Creative Living, for your wholehearted belief in my work. And last but not least, thank you Janet Mills and Gina Misiroglu for your editorial instincts, insight, patience, and attention to detail. You make being edited almost pleasant.

Contents

1

Getting Started

When I first heard about yoga, I was probably like most of the Western population. A part of me dwelled on the image of half-naked yogis folding themselves into human pretzels, another part conjured up serene thoughts of modern-day swamis, incense, and a kind of New Age spirituality. Through experience and discovery I quickly realized that neither of these images was correct. Yoga may be a centuries-old Eastern philosophy and art practiced by a variety of cultures, but it is also the finest, most adaptable form of combined physical and mental refreshment available today.

No longer confined to the realm of the mystic, yoga is shedding its exotic image and becoming recognized as a practical, powerful system of mind/body exercise appropriate for any age, any time frame. Medical establishments are using yoga to help prevent heart disease and treat injuries. Conservative businesses are integrating yoga into their daily course of events to manage stress and improve workplace productivity. Fitness instructors and mental health experts are advocating yoga as the practice of choice for busy business people who want to calm their minds, regenerate their bodies, and manage their lives with greater ease and joy. Yoga has taken its rightful place at the helm of today's busy and sophisticated lifestyle. And for good reason — it works.

After sitting in front of a computer all day, you probably feel like your neck and shoulders could use some unwinding. Your mind could use a "mental reprieve," because those ten-minute coffee breaks just don't seem to de-stress you anymore. And your back is so knotted that even a hot bath won't ease the ache. With just fifteen minutes of dedication a day, you'll learn how yoga can help even the tightest neck and pinching lower back feel good again. The practice is explained in simple, no-nonsense terms, and illustrated with two posture sequences that take into account your many roles and packed schedule. A variety of suggestions is included to keep your motivation high and help you maintain your practice schedule. At the end of the book, you'll find a list of excellent reading material for further study and a table of commonly asked questions with associated page references. Gurus, swamis, and the pop counterculture aside, yoga will help you increase your energy and revive your body's youthful flexibility like no other form of exercise.

What's So Great About Yoga?

Despite its Indian roots, yoga is basically a non-denominational, holistic practice, made-to-order for the busy Western persona. Yoga is a Sanskrit term, roughly meaning "yoke, or union." Its definition implies its purpose: to unite the mind, body, and spirit to enhance health and improve the overall quality of life. This book is about the most recognizable form of yoga practice, Hatha yoga. Hatha means "sun" and "moon," suggesting that the healthy union of opposites — in this case, the mind and body — lead to strength, vitality, and peace of mind. Hatha yoga is concerned less with the quantity of physical movement than its quality. By regularly combining precise, sustained stretches with mental focus and deep breathing, you quiet your mind and refresh your body. This in turn frees your spirit, making you not only healthier and more relaxed, but also genuinely happier.

It Quiets Your Mind

Yoga has long been known to calm and quiet the mind, yet few people understand the physiological basis for this effect. Fear and its surrogate, anxiety, release hormones that perpetuate stress reactions such as shallow breathing, muscle tension, dilated pupils, and other aspects of the fight-or-flight response. These physiological responses in turn reinforce the catalyst, fear, perpetuating a cycle of stress. Yoga is a powerful counteragent to this troublesome buildup because it breaks the cycle, helping your busy mind to quiet its agitation. This emotionally stabilizing influence is making yoga the core of stress-management programs offered throughout the United States.

In a way, yoga is a style of meditation. Meditation is a mental discipline of focusing the mind upon one thing or activity, the purpose of which is to develop a transcendent sense of peace and a mindful clarity of thought. Meditation teaches you how to efficiently think and act without the burden of reactive thinking. People who meditate regularly are light of heart, not oppressed by the crescendo of self-doubt that plagues Western culture. They listen to their thoughts but aren't trapped by them. They become objective, creative thinkers with excellent concentration skills. As you quiet your mind through yoga postures, you're exercising a form of this mental discipline.

It Refreshes Your Body

Contrary to a common notion that yoga simply twists your body into obscure, meaningless shapes, its combination of physical postures, breathing methods, and awareness practices are exquisitely natural. They harmonize with your body's unique structure and fundamental physical capabilities. Yoga practitioners will tell you that they experience greatly increased mental and physical energy after a posture sequence.

Physical distress is often the result of improper movement, or lack of it. We're a society of people who sit improperly, move incorrectly, and perform potentially damaging repetitive tasks, all of which create muscular imbalances in our bodies. Our bodies are crying out for alignment. In classic yoga lore, this alignment facilitates the smooth flow of vital life energy (known as "prana" or "chi") through the muscles, bones, and soft tissues. Using postures and sustained stretches, yoga skillfully and methodically aligns your body, bringing your skeleton, muscles, and internal organs back into balance.

Yoga's deep breathing practices combat fatigue, lower blood pressure, and can even ward off asthma attacks. The stretching and strengthening exercises relieve muscle strains, prevent injuries, lubricate joints, and increase endurance. In essence, yoga is the ultimate body tune-up.

As Jean Couch says in her excellent book, *The Runner's Yoga Book*, "I want you to know that if you follow a yoga program you will probably feel much better, better in a way that's hard to describe, because of the skeletal extension and muscular flexibility you will gain. Actually, I can think of a way to describe how you probably will feel: younger."

It Frees Your Spirit

Treasures such as peace of mind, joy, and contentment are often difficult to come by in today's harried world. Moments of potential quiet are inundated with appointments, responsibilities, and incessant mental chatter. Busy people long for the freedom that accompanies inner peace, but they don't know how to slow down, relax, and listen to the still, small voice inside.

Yoga helps ease your mind and soothe your body so that the connection to inner peace can be re-established. In this connection, your creative spirit can take flight into new ideas and expressions. You discover a calmness and emotional grace that lasts far longer than the length of the sequence. Mental chatter begins to subside as you explore the posture sequences. Your spirit is no longer hampered by physical and mental exhaustion or neurotic fear. You feel serene, clear-headed, and light-hearted.

The Busy Person's Advantage

You may believe that your busy lifestyle is a disadvantage when it comes to starting a practice such as yoga, but a full schedule of activity is actually helpful because it cultivates characteristics necessary to the development and maintenance of a vital yoga practice. These characteristics include curiosity, flexibility, and stamina.

1. *Curiosity*: Busy people tend to have a keen sense of curiosity. They ask questions and explore new ways to improve their efficiency. This is important because, as a yoga student, you are literally exploring your own mind and body. Your curiosity will spark a natural interest in yoga that will keep you from becoming complacent or bored with your practice.

2. *Flexibility*: Your full life demands an ability to shift gears and adapt. The world is constantly changing and, whether you like it or not, you have to be responsive and ready. This mental flexibility means that you can integrate and apply the positive character traits that yoga develops. Mental flexibility can also be directed into creative scheduling, helping you fit yoga into an already packed agenda.

3. *Stamina*: Keeping up a job, a social life, a family, and other responsibilities requires strength and endurance. If you can do all that, you can practice yoga. Because of your stamina and resilience, you won't give up on yoga even if the time constraints of your busy routine make

practice difficult.

In addition to having all the right qualities for starting a yoga practice, you also generate enough activity in your life to give you reason to continue yoga. The more activity in your world, the more opportunity you have to observe the benefits of yoga. With these benefits serving as motivation, you're much more likely to continue practicing.

What About Stress?

On a small scale, stress stimulates activity and improves concentration. This is one reason why college students often wait until the last minute to study for exams. The stress galvanizes their efforts so they can concentrate more easily.

Like college students, busy people tend to rely on stress to propel them through the gauntlet of distractions they confront every day. Unfortunately, requiring stress to get you going is like becoming ill to get attention. The end result is habitual sickness. Life becomes an endless series of dramas. Special events are forgotten. Weekdays and weekends fuse into one long jumble of responsibilities. Chronically stressed-out people believe that tomorrow is for living; today is for surviving.

Chronic mental stress not only affects your outlook on life, it also damages your body. Research has shown that it weakens your immune system, squeezes your coronary arteries, increases your blood pressure, shortens your breathing, and unduly tightens your muscles. It is a precursor to physical illness, particularly if you already have a family history of certain ailments like cancer or heart disease.

Cardiac specialists, psychoneuroimmunologists (people who study the relationship between the mind, the nervous system, and the immune system) and other medical and scientific professionals are now proving what yogis have known for generations: stretching the body, breathing deeply, oxygenating the brain, and lengthening the skeleton all lead to clear thinking, physical health, and stress reduction. With regular practice, yoga develops an emotional equanimity that increases your stress tolerance. People who've been practicing yoga say things like, "I just don't get upset like I used to. It takes a lot more to set me off."

You'll never have a stress-free life. Stress is an irrevocable part of the human equation. However, you can learn to cope with stress effectively and keep it from building a permanent residence in your mind and body. Yoga, the contemporary 2000-year-old practice, will teach you how.

Finding the Correct Style

Yoga styles vary from flowing, moving forms that demand certain strength levels, to long, slow processes of holding postures steady for periods of time. While all styles are beneficial, the Yoga for Busy People method employs a style that's perfect for busy people because of its focus on precision and accuracy. It helps you glean the most value from every movement in every posture.

Yoga's birthplace is India. As such, it was originally developed for Indian bodies accustomed to postures and activities very different from those we encounter in North America. The Western lifestyle doesn't make our bodies strong and flexible in the same way that Indian bodies are strong and flexible. Hence, at first, you may need props such as yoga mats, pillows, belts, and chairs to help you achieve the correct alignment. This is natural, expected, and doesn't mean yoga is wrong for you.

To know if a yoga style is proper for you, tune into your body and listen to its responses. If you are new to yoga, if your body is inflexible or overweight, or if you have physical limitations, give yourself time to mature into the poses. Ask yourself how you feel after a yoga session. Do you feel refreshed, invigorated, alive? If not, then you may need to slow down or investigate another exercise form.

Because every body is different, you may need to personalize your sequence once you understand the correct execution of the movements and their ultimate aims. Further study and attention to how your body feels will tell you whether or not certain postures are appropriate for you. However, you'll never know what yoga can do for you unless you try it for at least three weeks. If you're consistent in your practice, three weeks of effort will tell you if yoga can make a difference in your life. I'm betting that it can, and that you'll begin to feel comfortable with this newfound exercise program after a few short practice sessions.

The Yoga for Busy People Method

The Yoga for Busy People (YBP) method addresses issues that busy people often contend with — little time, little physical flexibility, and a crowded mind. It offers a logical order of progression, leaving enough room for variety but not straying far from the desired result — maximum value in a minimal amount of time. Here is a brief overview of YBP's three simple steps:

1. *Center your attention*: Centering refines your concentration and quiets your mind. Centering cultivates a keen awareness of what your body is doing. It teaches your mind to focus, attunes your attention to the body's alignment and

breathing rhythm, and intensifies the value of any posture. As the first part of any yoga session, centering prepares you mentally and emotionally for your postures.

2. *Perform a posture*: When you execute a yoga posture or a series of postures as described in Chapters 2 and 4 of this book, you'll be concentrating on a specific part of your body, while refreshing your body overall. Each posture aligns, tones, lengthens, and nourishes your muscles and internal organs. It's more beneficial to correctly execute a single posture than to thoughtlessly run through a series of postures.

3. *Release the experience*: Releasing involves accepting what you've done and letting go of the experience. Releasing reinforces the value of the practice, enhancing its long-term effect. With an upbeat, positive release, you're also less likely to procrastinate your next practice session.

Properly executed, these three steps turn any stretch, posture, or series of postures into an experience which is body-invigorating, stress-reducing, and mind-refreshing. Overlooking a step may weaken the value of the practice, turning it into just another stretching session.

As you experience these three steps, remember that yoga is done with a combination of flow and accuracy. You don't simply bounce into a pose. You consciously move every part of your being into it. This attention to detail makes you intensely aware of all your body's moving parts — their exquisite precision, their strengths, their frailties. You learn how to re-inhabit your body instead of ignoring or dismissing it. You develop a childlike partnership with your body that is both freeing and energy producing.

How Long Should You Practice?

If you're wondering how to motivate yourself to fit yoga into a very short time frame (see Chapters 3 and 4), then you'll probably need to think about scheduling time for it. Ideally, you should practice some form of yoga daily for a minimum of fifteen to twenty minutes, with a couple of thirty-minute sessions each week. (Think of daily yoga as a quick, invigorating mind/body shower.) Of course, asking you to add yet another daily "have-to" to your already overextended schedule may be too much. So if you can't create a regular routine, do yoga whenever you can for as long as you can. Hopefully you can squeeze a minimum of four fifteen-minute practice sessions into a week. The main point is: *do it*. Do it whenever you think about it. If you only have time for one posture, do one posture. Don't deny yourself the value of a single posture just because you don't have time for a whole sequence. Yoga makes you feel so good that you'll find yourself naturally carving out more time for it.

In a regular practice schedule, the following breakdown of times is recommended for beginners:

1. *For centering your attention*: Start with one or two minutes, then increase as you feel the inclination.

2. *For performing a posture*: This depends on the posture or series of postures. You can do a single standing posture for as little as thirty

seconds, or a series of postures lasting up to thirty minutes. Fifteen minutes is a good start for a busy beginner.

3. *For releasing the experience*: One or two minutes.

If you tend to hurry through your postures, then you're treating yoga like any other form of exercise and your results will be less than optimal. You may improve your muscle tone, but inwardly you'll still be overwrought and exhausted. Eventually you'll probably lose interest, returning to your uptight, physically constricted, stressed-out condition. Rushing through yoga is like rowing a boat with only one oar in the water: You generate a lot of speed but you don't get anywhere.

When I find myself rushing into yoga, I play a game. I say, "I'm going to not hurry for fifteen minutes. That's all. Fifteen minutes of not hurrying isn't going to make me late. When the fifteen minutes are up, I'll hurry again." If I have a choice between rushing through six poses or correctly executing two poses, I only do two. I move slowly and breathe deeply through the postures. When my sequence is complete, I'm not only stretched and strengthened, I'm also relaxed, alert, and ready to move on. Even though I give myself the opportunity to continue hurrying when my fifteen minutes are up, I usually choose not to. Hurrying is no longer necessary because my mind is clear and therefore I'm more alert and efficient.

Creating the Right Environment

Yoga isn't limited to specific locations or environmental conditions. In a perfect world, however, it is best to do yoga in a temperate location where you can be focused. You don't have to be alone, but you should be able to minimize distracting sounds and intrusions. Your exercise surface should be smooth and level, and your attire should be nonrestrictive.

1. *Find a temperate location.* Like other forms of exercise, yoga generates heat and sweat. Unlike other forms of exercise, yoga includes quiet

nonmoving segments that may make you cold. I handle these concerns by keeping the room temperate (67 to 75 degrees) and layering a couple of T-shirts, which I can pull off and on as necessary. I also keep a blanket handy for the release portion of the sequence, because when I lie still I sometimes get a little chilly.

If you do your practice outside, try to find a level spot with plenty of room for stretching and balancing. Dress accordingly; if it's cold, wear more layers.

2. *Keep your focus.* You don't have to be physically alone, but you do need to create a quiet space in your mind. If the dogs and kids distract you from your quiet mind, you might try doing yoga while they're asleep or playing outside. If you practice with a friend or partner, try to keep from talking while you move through the postures. This is your special time to connect with your inner self. Interacting with someone else can disrupt this process.

3. *Minimize distractions.* Yoga is best performed with the natural sounds of your environment.

Ideally, those natural sounds are hushed in order to minimize distraction. If you use background music, keep it soft and "meditative." (Refer to Chapter 3.) Similarly, distracting noises such as the television, telephone, and answering machine should be kept to a minimum.

4. *Find a level surface.* It's nice to have a bare floor available because carpets don't always provide enough traction. If you're working out on a bare floor, use a mat to cushion your body. (You can make your own yoga mat or you can mail order it.) I do yoga on my kitchen floor. It's a wood floor so it doesn't get too cold, and my bare feet can get a good grip on the finish.

   If you're doing yoga outdoors, most any surface is appropriate as long as it's level and you feel comfortable sitting or lying on it. I prefer grass to concrete for obvious reasons, but any surface will do.

5. *Wear comfortable clothing.* A nonrestrictive, breathable material such as cotton is appropriate for yoga as long as the clothing is warm but not bulky. You'll find that bare feet (as opposed

to socks) make the postures a little easier to maintain because of the traction bare skin creates. The less material between the soles of your feet and the workout surface, the more sensitive you'll be to posture, balance, and alignment. You want to maximize your sense of connection to the ground. If you're outdoors, any soft, flat-soled shoe will do.

A word of advice: If you can't create an ideal environment, don't worry about it. I've done yoga in airports, cars, and dental offices. As you read through this book and explore the various postures, you'll find your own creative ways to fit yoga into your busy lifestyle.

The Expectation Trap

The problem with starting any new discipline is that it's difficult to differentiate between a motivating vision and an impossible standard. With yoga, you could paper your walls with pictures of strong, often young, lithe bodies folded into advanced postures. These pictures are meant to be instructive and motivating. Unfortunately, they frequently serve the opposite function.

"I can't do what those athletes can do," laments a 60-year-old beginning yoga student as she stares at the photos. "I've got back trouble and there's no way I can even touch my toes. Maybe this is something you have to start at a young age." A young man recovering from knee surgery complains, "With my knee, I'm never going to be able to get into those deep bending postures. If I can't do it right, I don't want to do it at all." An overweight student wonders if she even belongs in a yoga class. "How can I compare myself to these people?" she says, pointing to the photos. "Maybe I should do something else."

Each of these beginners started yoga with high hopes; each fell head first into the expectation trap. That is, they compared themselves to advanced practitioners and decided they couldn't measure up. Instead of deriving hope from their role models, they used them as excuses to quit. A yoga instructor describes it this way: "Students begin yoga with great expectations. But yoga involves listening to and observing your body. For some people, this is the first time they've looked directly at their tension, their weak muscles, their shallow breathing. They don't expect to see themselves so clearly and it can be a little daunting. The excuses to quit surface pretty quickly."

The important thing to remember is that yoga must be personalized. Your body isn't like anyone else's body. Except for purposes of instruction, comparisons in yoga are folly. For you, a forward bend may be easy but a backward bend is impossible. For someone else, the opposite is true. Your slight lift into a partial backward bend is as powerful and useful to your body as a perfect backward bend is to the veteran student. Fulfillment in yoga is a game of inches, and the only inches that count are yours. As you inch slowly toward deeper, more advanced postures, you make an enormous difference in the health and flexibility of your body. Through minor successes your body reaps major rewards.

Further, every posture has an almost Infinite number of variations. These variations can accommodate almost any physical restriction. What matters is your positioning: If you're aligned in the posture, you receive the benefits. The expectation trap has no place in yoga. When you see it, steer clear.

Remember that yoga is much more than physical flexibility and strength. In the classic sense, it is a way to unify our minds through the mechanism of our bodies. The mental work you do with each posture — centering, observing, releasing — adds emotional equanimity and balance to your life. You are developing internal skills that can't be measured by how far you bend.

Now you're ready to begin!

2

Your Yoga Program

The complete YBP program is made up of many components. Fundamental to the program are three simple steps that form the foundation of meaningful yoga practice. These steps help you organize any group of postures into an effective practice sequence that will fit into any time frame and ensure that you'll derive the most benefit from your daily yoga routine. To help you prepare for yoga and maximize the value of each posture, you'll find a list of tips — keys to effective practice — which are meant to accent the yoga steps, enriching your practice time. At first, it may seem difficult to juggle these new techniques together, but soon the steps and tips will feel natural and easy to incorporate into the posture sequences.

The second half of this chapter presents two posture sequences that are relatively quick, easy to remember, and thorough. These sequences are only suggestions; once you learn the basics you can reorganize the order of the postures to suit your own personal preferences and time constraints. Ultimately, the combination of the three simple steps, the keys to effective practice, and the two posture sequences synthesize into a simple, effective yoga program designed to cull the greatest benefit from the smallest time frame.

YBP's Three Simple Steps

The three simple steps that comprise the YBP program serve as the basis for any posture sequence you perform. Though the second half of this chapter provides you with two complete posture sequences, you may not always have the time or suitable conditions to perform every part of them. As a busy person, you'll need to quickly build a sequence of postures that fit within the constraints of your schedule. The three steps outlined here will not only help you organize an effective posture combination, they will help you derive the most benefit from the postures you choose. The three basic steps are as follows: 1) center your attention, 2) perform the posture(s), and 3) release the experience.

Step 1: Center Your Attention

You've probably driven your car and upon arrival at your destination realized you couldn't remember the details of driving there. Your driving responses were on auto-pilot, your mind a thousand miles away. The same thing can happen with yoga. You can perform all the postures without being mentally present. This turns yoga into just another stretch routine — boring, limited, poorly executed, and easily avoided. To derive the greatest benefit from yoga, your attention should be focused on your body's messages as it moves through each posture sequence. This is accomplished through mental centering.

Centering is a process of becoming in tune with the present moment. When you center, you pay attention to one thing such as your breathing, the sensations in your body, or a phrase or prayer. Your focus is sharp, clear, and without preconception. In yoga, centering helps you respond quickly and intelligently to your body's messages. It also refreshes your mind and strengthens your concentration. This helps you remain alert and composed long after the posture sequence is completed.

Initially, centering may seem somewhat foreign, but you'll find that it becomes easier as you practice it. I occasionally use a set of words that help me remain attentive yet relaxed.

Breathe in, and say to yourself "in."
Breathe out, and say to yourself "out."
Breathe in, and say to yourself "deep."
Breathe out, and say to yourself "soft."
Breathe in, and say to yourself "here."
Breathe out, and say to yourself "now."

The first step in your yoga program is center ing your attention. Begin by scanning the sensations in your body from the bottoms of your feet to the top of your head. Your attention should be sharp, clear, and without negative judgment. If you detect discomfort or stress, gently adjust your body position until you feel stable and relaxed, your weight evenly balanced. (For more details about scanning your body, refer to the Bottom-to-Top Alignment Scan, later in this chapter.) When the body scan is complete, briefly focus on your breathing. For two or three breathing cycles (one inhalation and one exhalation form one cycle), pay attention to your breath as you draw it in and let it out. Don't try to make it do anything. Just observe and feel it. If your attention strays, bring it back to the moment, back to the breathing process.

Though "formal" centering ends with the beginning of the posture sequence, you should continue to center your attention on the postures themselves. The beauty of yoga is that you are centering on a body that is moving, stretching, always changing. Instead of thinking about the details of your business meeting, your mind can attend to the tension in your knee or the extra stretch in your hamstring while smiling, breathing, strengthening, and relaxing.

Step 2: Perform a Posture

Once you're physically and mentally centered, you're ready to perform a posture or a sequence of postures. The suggested YBP posture sequences are divided into two groups: standing and floor sequences. Standing postures are invigorating and strengthening; they teach you principles of correct movement and carriage. Floor postures are calming to the mind and soothing to the nerves; they promote healthy sleep. It's best to learn the postures in their proper sequence before mixing and matching them.

Each posture should be held for a minimum of two breathing cycles. It's also helpful to repeat postures in which you feel particularly stiff in order to explore them more deeply. You might want to come back to an earlier pose because your body feels looser toward the end of the sequence.

As you read through the posture descriptions, you may find certain instructions to be unfamiliar, such as keeping your back *long* and your tailbone *down*. These instructions allude to the body stretching in opposite directions. Every posture should be performed with the image that the head and the feet are extending away from the center of the body. The idea is to elongate your body without flattening or swaying your back, and lengthen your spine without over- or under-tucking your pelvis. Imagine two silken cords connected to your spine: one is attached to your neck and the other is attached to your tailbone. Visualize these two cords gently pulling in opposite directions, elongating your spine in harmony with its natural structure and alignment.

Approach the postures with respect and curiosity. Using your centered awareness, observe the sensations as you stretch into a pose. Listen to the messages your body is sending. If an area is inflexible, make a mental note to give it more attention. A posture that you perform poorly could be exactly what your body needs to practice. Listen to your muscles and joints, not your ego.

Step 3: Release the Experience

Deep relaxation and release work is integral to yoga. Releasing frees you from the event and helps you move forward. In a positive sense, you make peace with the results of the experience even if they aren't as remarkable as you would like. Releasing keeps you from overanalyzing your performance by saying, "I did the best I could under the circumstances. I'm ready to let the experience go and move on."

In yoga, releasing is more than a mental practice; it's enhanced by restful poses that conclude a posture sequence. Oftentimes, yoga students faithfully execute a sequence of postures but neglect to enjoy the exquisite rejuvenation that flows from the deep relaxation. After a deep relaxation, release is simple. The mind and body, refreshed and revitalized, are ready to move into the next activity with restored energy and enthusiasm.

Releasing also prepares you to repeat the experience, bolstered by positive expectancy. Instead of fueling feelings of inadequacy or dread, release work celebrates your intention and effort, regardless of your actual performance. The fact that you even showed up to do yoga is a success.

It's important to remember these three steps as you become proficient at creating personalized posture sequences. Always begin by centering, then perform the postures, and finally release the experience as positive and useful. As you practice the steps, you'll begin to see how they apply to each individual posture as well as the full sequence. For example, before the Supine Hamstring Stretch (page 79), you breathe to center awareness in your body, then lift into the posture and sustain it for a few breaths, then return to neutral and release the stretch as a success. You let it go with a breath and move to the next posture.

Keys to Effective Practice

Yoga is more than just body exercise; it's *mind/body* exercise. Yoga teachers remind their students of this by coaching them to take note of the messages their bodies convey as they perform each posture. To help you cultivate this mind/body awareness and to substantially enrich your experience of yoga, study and apply the following keys to effective practice. These keys may not replace the coaching of a good yoga teacher, but they'll help maximize the pleasure, safety, and efficacy of the yoga posture sequences.

Learn to Breathe with Your Abdomen

A combination of poor posture, long hours behind desks, and flat-stomach phobia turns many Westerners into "chest breathers" — people who expand only the upper chest when they inhale. Chest breathing is akin to partially filling a car's gasoline tank. The car works, but it's always running on empty. Chest breathing can also exacerbate breathlessness by creating an imbalance in the oxygen/carbon dioxide ratio, which results in hyperventilation and dizziness.

Deep abdominal breathing promotes a full

exchange of air, keeping the oxygen/carbon diox
ide ratio balanced. It opens the lungs. It dispels fatigue and anxiety. It feels delicious. Most important, it nourishes the muscles and organs with
oxygen, helping you relax deeply and safely into a
posture. To know if you're breathing abdominally,
simply place your hands over your stomach and
inhale. If the stomach expands when you inhale
and contracts when you exhale, that's good. If your
chest expands but your stomach does not, then
you're chest breathing. Practice expanding your
stomach when you inhale, not just your chest.

Breathe Naturally and Without Force

Even though other forms of yoga employ
rhythmic or forced breathing patterns, the YBP
program advocates breathing easily, naturally, and
abdominally. Inhale and exhale through the nose
without forcing any particular tempo (except
where it is specified in the posture description).
Natural breathing is appropriate for busy people
attempting to squeeze a stretch or posture into the

work day with the least amount of fuss. My only suggestion is that you use the execution of the posture as a framework for inhaling and exhaling. Generally speaking, inhale in preparation for a posture and exhale as you move into it. If you're performing a series of postures, try resting between each pose for at least one inhale/exhale breathing cycle unless otherwise instructed.

Do a Bottom-to-Top Alignment Scan

Good pilots extol the importance of pre-flight checks. A pre-flight check is a systematic, orderly scan of the plane's fuel mixture, engine condition, and structural integrity. These scans ensure that the foundations for a safe flight are all in place.

Just as the plane is the vehicle for the pilot, so the body is the vehicle for the yoga student. If you have an unbalanced foundation, you may not be strengthening or stretching the appropriate muscles and could have trouble maintaining postures. The bottom-to-top alignment scan is a form of pre-flight check because it ensures that your vehicle foundation is balanced and stable, from the bottoms of your feet to the top of your head.

Here's how to do an alignment scan when you perform a standing posture sequence. Stand straight and tall, starting your scan at the bottom — the foundation — of your body, the feet and legs. Make sure your ankles aren't rolling in and that your weight is evenly distributed between both feet. As you examine your knees and hips, make sure the knees are sturdy but not locked and that the tailbone is moving down to avoid a sway back. Next, pay attention to your stomach and chest, breathing abdominally and lifting everything up from the hip bones. Notice your back and spine, feeling them elongate. Roll your shoulders gently back and down, feeling your collarbone broaden. Let your arms drop loosely against your sides and continue scanning up your neck, lifting from the crown of the head to extend the spine. Keep your chin level, take another deep breath, and exhale, releasing any undue tension from the throat and face. Smile — you're doing a great job!

The bottom-to-top alignment scan can also be

done when you perform a floor sequence. Simply sit comfortably and go through the same bottom-to-top steps. You may initially have to teach yourself how a strong foundation feels. With a little practice, however, you'll be able to align bottom-to-top anywhere, in any position, in less than a minute.

Don't Bounce into a Posture

Yoga postures are sustained stretches. In yoga you are attempting to lengthen the resting state of your muscles and tendons. Bouncing into a stretch does little to lengthen the muscle spindle and it may even contribute to shortening and tightening your muscles. Further, bouncing a tense muscle can cause it to strain or tear.

Never Strain Your Muscles

Stretching is beneficial; straining is harmful. With yoga, you're attempting to challenge your body, not attack it. If you push too hard, you'll weaken or injure your body instead of helping it become stronger. Yoga walks a mindful line between complacency and assertiveness. If you're not sure whether you're doing beneficial stretching or harmful straining, look at how you habitually approach exercise. If you tend to overextend, be more careful and take it slowly. If you tend to baby yourself, be more adventurous and push a little. Regardless, the best way to avoid straining is to stretch until you feel the muscle pull, then ease up just a little and remain in the stretch. If you do the posture again, you'll probably find that you can stretch a little farther into it.

Smile As You Do the Posture

Most people wear taut, unyielding facial expressions when they concentrate or learn something new. This tension takes a toll on facial muscles, leading to permanently furrowed brows and other unwelcome character lines. But more important, facial tension is a sign that tension is running throughout the body.

Facial tension is common among yoga students

because they're always learning new postures, stretching tense muscles, and trying very hard to do everything right. Fortunately, facial tension can change with a smile. Natural smiling releases tension. Smiling triggers feelings of generosity, pleasure, and relaxation. It lightens the feigned seriousness of the yoga sequence. As you practice your yoga, remind yourself to smile. Your face and body will respond more easily to the movements.

If It Hurts Too Much, Stop

Discomfort doesn't always mean you're doing something wrong. Stretching very tight muscles, such as hamstrings, can be somewhat uncomfortable until you're used to it. However, you must never let discomfort go unattended. Let the discomfort speak to you. Is it telling you that the movement is inappropriate for your body? Is it telling you to do a less-advanced version of the pose? Is it telling you to slow down and rest?

Use the BS, BT Reminder

The Breathe, Smile, Bottom-to-Top (BS, BT) reminder is a simple formula designed to maximize the value you receive from each yoga posture as you perform it. BS, BT serves as an easy-to-remember guide to help you slow down and focus on the posture(s) you're doing. This is particularly important if you only have time to do one or two postures. Briefly, BS, BT reminds you to:

1) Breath abdominally to relax and regenerate your body.
2) Smile to release tension and lighten your attitude.
3) Scan your body from the bottoms of your feet to the top of your head to assure proper balance and alignment within the posture. (Refer to page 46.)

As you step through the posture sequences, use BS, BT to keep you on track. Regardless of your time constraints, this approach will help you get the most out of each posture.

Check with Your Doctor

Yoga is not meant to be a substitute for your doctor. In fact, physical therapists, medical doctors, and chiropractors often prescribe yoga to help their patients recover from injuries or surgery. If you have any limiting physical conditions such as arthritis, back problems, or chronic injuries, you should check with your doctor before starting this or any other exercise program.

The Posture Sequences

A posture sequence is a progression of yoga "exercises," ideally organized around YBP's three simple steps. Each posture (also known by the Sanskrit term, *asana*) is a carefully conceived pose whose every movement is designed to strengthen, tone, and condition the body inside and out. Yoga teachers develop posture sequences based on their philosophies, educational backgrounds, and life experiences. As the teachers grow and change, they sometimes change the order of postures or enhance them in personally meaningful ways.

With literally hundreds of variations, there is an unending variety of postures, or poses, to string together. Different yoga styles execute these postures in diverse ways. Some styles advocate moving quickly from one posture to the next; other styles stress the precision of slow movement and sustained stretches. Some styles include jumping, others include intensive breathing practices. The two posture sequences defined in this book — the standing sequence and the floor sequence — offer a little of everything. The standing sequence is a flowing, almost aerobic experience while the floor sequence is slower and more restful.

The postures involved in the two sequences described below are basic; use this guide as an introduction to them. If you're more experienced with yoga, these sequence descriptions can help to maintain the precision of your practice. Keep in mind that yoga postures have many modifications depending on your flexibility, skill level, and body condition. It never hurts to expand your posture repertoire by reading other yoga books or renting videos. (See Appendix 1 for a list of excellent reference books and tapes.) Another option is to find a good yoga teacher and start classes. But even if you can't find a class in your area, this book will get you started on the right track.

Sequence 1: The Standing Sequence

Standing postures are energizing, strengthening, and invigorating. If you're drowsy at your desk or daydreaming when you should be concentrating, a standing yoga sequence can wake you up, enliven your body and circulation, and ready you for productive activity.

The order of execution (using YBP's three simple steps) is as follows: 1) center your attention with Shoulder Rolls and Neck Stretches; 2) perform the standing postures of the Warrior and the Sun Salutation; and 3) release the experience with the Corpse.

Begin the sequence by centering your mind. Scan your body, bottom-to-top, making sure your weight is properly balanced and aligned. Use the

BS, BT reminder to relax and attend to your body's messages, movements, and the natural flow of the breath. Complete the centering process with Shoulder Rolls and Neck Stretches. These movements relax and support body alignment, preparing you for the ensuing postures.

Shoulder Rolls

Shoulder Rolls are simple, powerful centering exercises that can be performed anywhere. They help you unwind by loosening tight muscles in your neck and shoulders, and stretching your upper chest and back. As you center your attention on the Shoulder Rolls, observe the movement of the joints, the opening of the chest and back, and the lifting of the neck.

How:

1. Stand (or sit) up straight, arms at your sides. Lift your head up from the crown, gently elongating the neck.

2. With your arms hanging loose at your sides, roll the shoulders forward (fig. 2-1a), up to

the ears (fig. 2-1b), back to the center of the back (fig. 2-1c), and down. Do this a couple of times, breathing naturally. Then repeat in the opposite direction.

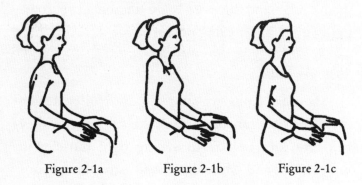

Figure 2-1a   Figure 2-1b   Figure 2-1c

Remember:

* Use the muscles in your upper back, chest, and shoulders. Don't use your arms.
* Visualize your neck remaining loose and soft; otherwise it might tense up in an effort to help the shoulders do their work.

Neck Stretches

Neck Stretches are just as simple, powerful, and adaptable as Shoulder Rolls. They're an excellent centering activity because the movements are small and the neck is sensitive. It's a good idea to perform Neck Stretches after Shoulder Rolls because your muscles will be a little more limber and flexible. As you center your attention on the neck, observe the differences in flexibility from one side of the neck to the other. Notice your tendency to want to stretch "a little farther."

Figure 2-2b

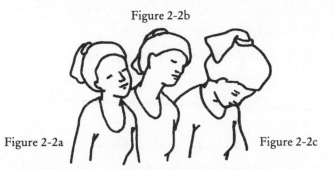

Figure 2-2a   Figure 2-2c

How:

1. Stand (or sit) up straight, arms at your sides. Lift your head up from the crown, gently elongating the neck.

2. With your arms hanging loose at your sides, your chin level and eyes looking straight ahead, bend your right ear toward your right

shoulder (fig. 2-2a). Hold for at least one breathing cycle, then lift your head back to center.

3. Keep your chin level, eyes looking forward, and bend your left ear toward your left shoulder (fig. 2-2b). Hold for at least one breathing cycle and return to center.

4. Let your head hang forward, your chin next to your chest (fig. 2-2c). Hold for one breathing cycle and return to center.

5. Repeat the above Neck Stretches at least one more time.

Remember:

* Keep your chin level to offset the tendency to collapse your head back. The idea is to drop your ear straight down toward your shoulder, eyes looking forward.

* Let gravity pull your ear toward your shoulder. Don't try to force it. Relax into the stretch.

* Don't stretch your shoulder up to meet your ear. Keep the other shoulder relaxed and

down. The shoulders should be low and loose, the chest broad.

The Warrior

The Warrior is a vigorous posture, filling the body with strength. It stretches the muscles of the legs and ankles, opens the chest and groin, and stimulates the entire body. It also develops balance and stamina. The Warrior is excellent to perform at the beginning of a yoga sequence or by itself as a quick break from work.

How:

1. Stand facing forward with your feet as wide apart as is comfortable. Your legs are strong, the pelvis is tucked in slightly, and the crown of your head stretches easily up from the shoulders.
2. Stretch your arms out to the sides, parallel to the floor, palms down. Feel your collarbone broaden as your hands move away from each other (fig. 2-3a).
3. Inhale. Turn your left foot out 90 degrees

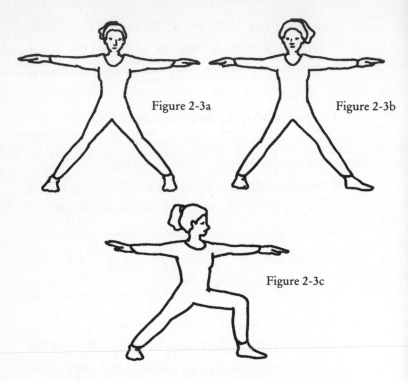

Figure 2-3a   Figure 2-3b

Figure 2-3c

and your right foot in the same direction up
to about 15 degrees (fig. 2-3b).

4. Exhale. Bend your left leg into a right angle
   so that the knee is directly over your ankle.
   (No farther!) Press your right heel into the
   floor to help steady you. Keep your left

ankle from rolling in on itself. Turn your head and look over your left arm (fig. 2-3c). Hold the position for one to three breathing cycles.

5. Repeat with the opposite leg.

Modifications:

* If you have difficulty maintaining alignment, try doing the Warrior alongside of a wall.
* If your back leg needs support, place your heel against a floor board and push into it as you extend into the pose.

Remember:

* Do not bend your knee beyond a right angle; it places undue strain on the knee joint.
* Keep your tailbone down as you step into the position. Your body should remain aligned and straight. Keep lifting up, not over.
* Use the strength of your legs to move back to a starting position.

The Sun Salutation

The Sun Salutation is a set of yoga postures performed in a nonstop linear fashion. The beauty of the Sun Salutation is that it stretches, strengthens, and challenges every part of your body in one graceful series. Each position counteracts the previous one, expanding and contracting your torso and regulating your breathing. The Sun Salutation can be performed slowly or more quickly — dispelling the notion that yoga doesn't elevate your heart rate. As you become more comfortable with the movements, they take on a satisfying, dance-like elegance.

The Sun Salutation sequence should be performed twice; first leading with the left foot (Step 3), and second leading with the right foot. A good way to learn the Sun Salutation is to take it in segments. Depending on your comfort level, do only the first three or four movements for a few days. When you have them memorized, add a new movement each day or whenever it feels appropriate and safe to do so. Ideally, you should synchronize your movements with your breathing. And don't avoid the tougher movements — they're showing you areas that need work and attention.

How:

1. Stand solid, weight evenly balanced over both feet, arms loose at your sides. Inhale, stretch your arms straight up, bending back slightly (fig. 2-4a/b).

2. Exhale, bend over from the hips, reaching your hands out to your sides and then down toward the floor. Bend as far as you comfortably can, no more (fig. 2-4c).

3. Inhale. If necessary, bend your knees to place your hands flat on the floor, on either side of your feet. Stretch the left foot back and try to keep the right knee bent in a 90-degree angle (fig. 2-4d). If necessary, drop the left knee to the ground to help support you.

4. Exhale. Stretch the right foot back to join the left foot. Lift your hips and thighs up and back, your weight still evenly balanced

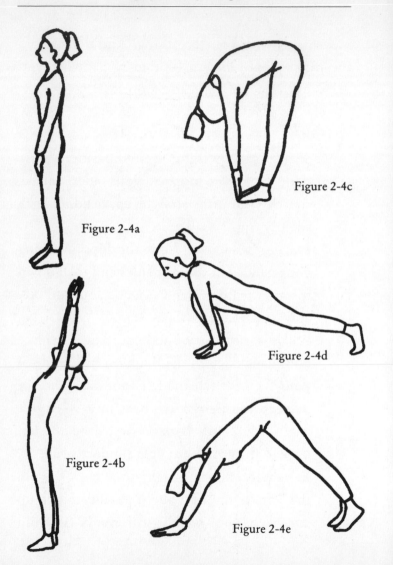

Figure 2-4a

Figure 2-4b

Figure 2-4c

Figure 2-4d

Figure 2-4e

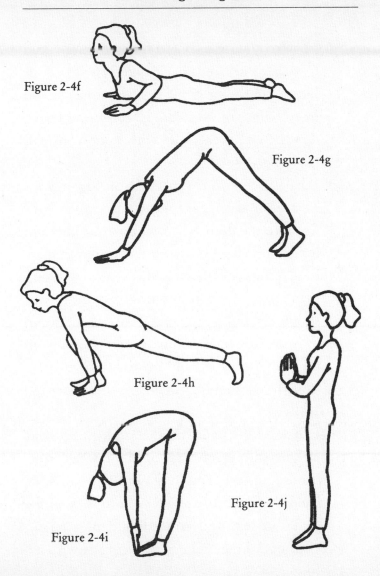

Figure 2-4f

Figure 2-4g

Figure 2-4h

Figure 2-4i

Figure 2-4j

between your hands and feet. You may need to walk your hands back slightly to get your hips up in the air. Your legs and arms should be straight, your back long, your head facing down on an even plane with your arms and back (fig. 2-4e).

5. Inhale. Bend your arms as you lower your hips even with your head, dropping your knees to the floor followed by your hips and torso. Straighten out your body, toes to forehead (arms still bent and supporting you), then press up with your arms until your shoulders and upper chest are off the floor, eyes looking forward, not down. Don't bend up from the waist, only from the upper back. Your naval should remain on the floor (fig. 2-4f).

6. Exhale. Lift your hips straight up, your weight still evenly balanced between your hands and feet. You may need to walk your hands back slightly to get your hips up in the air. Your legs and arms should be straight, your back long, your head facing down on a

even plane with your arms and back (fig. 2-4g).

7. Inhale. Bring the left foot forward between the hands (or as close as you can), attempting to keep the knee bent in a 90-degree angle. You may need to scoot your foot up between your hands (fig. 2-4h). If necessary, drop the right knee to the ground to help support you.

8. Exhale. Bring the right foot up to join the left foot. Straighten your legs as much as possible, with your body folded over at the hips (fig. 2-4i).

9. Inhale. Roll gently up with your arms at your sides, using your stomach to support you. Stretch your arms up over your head and bend back slightly, then straighten and lower your hands into a prayer position at the middle of the chest (fig. 2-4j).

Remember:

* Patience is the key. This isn't a flexibility competition. Your body has to be gently

introduced to the movements, and it may take time to develop enough strength to rhythmically coordinate moving and breathing.

* If you find certain movements too taxing, then modify the sequence to exclude them or do them in a manner your body can handle.

The Corpse

The Corpse is good for relaxing and releasing your yoga experience. The name isn't meant to be morbid; it's an image of stillness. (For details on release work, refer to page 42, Release the Experience.)

The Corpse involves more than just lying on your back (fig. 2-5). As many of you know, lying flat can be uncomfortable. Take the time to adjust your position so that all parts of your body feel completely supported and at ease. Have a few pillows handy in case you need some extra support under your knees or head. Since you may become cold as your circulation quiets down, keep a sweater or blanket close at hand.

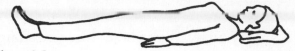

Figure 2-5

How:

1. Lie on your back with your legs straight and your arms slightly out from your body. Support the back of your head and upper neck with a blanket or pillow.

2. To help relax your back, pull your shoulder blades in toward your spine and then release them. Lift your knees up slightly, flatten your lower back to the floor, then slowly lower your knees keeping the tailbone comfortably extended.

3. Close your eyes and breathe naturally. Let your body weight sink into the floor. Allow your mind to settle, letting it gently note the body sensations or observe your breathing cycles. Remain lying on your back for two to five minutes, or longer if you prefer.

4. To end the Corpse, slowly open and close your eyes until they easily remain open, then

turn over on your side. Whenever you're ready, use your hands to help you sit upright.

Modifications:

* If your back is bothering you, prop your lower legs up on a chair or place a few pillows underneath your knees. You can also bend your knees and lean them against each other, with your feet about shoulder-length apart. This will help relieve stress in your lumbar spine. Explore whatever support is necessary for your body to feel completely relaxed.

Remember:

* The idea is not to sleep, but to relax deeply. If you find yourself beginning to sleep, try attending more carefully to your body sensations.
* As you relax, acknowledge yourself for taking the time to do yoga. Good work!

Sequence 2: The Floor Sequence

Floor postures are restful and soothing. They effectively stretch the body without requiring your legs to keep you balanced and upright. If your back is achy or your hamstrings feel tight and sore, floor exercises can loosen the tension gently and pleasantly. If you're having problems sleeping, floor exercises can help you fall asleep naturally by calming your busy mind and minimizing the distraction of a tense body.

The order of execution (using YBP's three simple steps) is as follows: 1) center your attention with the Easy Pose; 2) perform the floor postures of the Downward-Facing Dog, the Cobra, the Supine Hamstring Stretch, and the Floor Twist; and 3) release the experience with the Pose of a Child.

As with the standing sequence, begin by centering your mind. In this case, sit in the Easy Pose before beginning your bottom-to-top body scan. Use the BS, BT reminder to relax and attend to your body's messages, movements, and the natural flow of the breath. Complete your centering in the Easy Pose before moving into the next postures.

The Easy Pose

The Easy Pose probably seems familiar to you; most people have experienced sitting in an uncomfortable cross-legged position at one time or another. Because the Easy Pose is meant to be comfortable, take advantage of pillows and blankets to support your knees and hips. Once you're at ease, center your attention by letting the floor fully support the weight of your body. Feel your knees relax, your hips and pelvis widen, and your upper body lift gently so that the chest is broad and the spine comfortably straight (fig. 2-6).

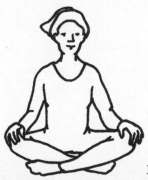

Figure 2-6

How:

1. Place a pillow (or folded blanket) on the floor, cross your legs, and sit on the edge of the pillow, weight balanced between your sitting bones, knees parallel to the floor.
2. Roll your shoulders forward, up to your ears, back to the center of the back, and drop them down. Keep your chin level, lifting up from the crown of the head. Rest your hands on your knees, arms loose at your sides (fig. 2-6). Keep lifting from the crown to eliminate hunching. Remain in this position until you've completed your centering practice.

Modifications:

* If you need extra support, sit with your back against a wall.
* If your hips are tight, support your knees with pillows.
* If the Easy Pose is impossible for you, sit in a straight-back chair or lie flat on the floor.

The Downward-Facing Dog

The Downward-Facing Dog stretches the back of the legs, the buttocks and back muscles, the shoulders and neck. It also strengthens and stretches the wrists and arms. It's a perfect, all-around posture that elongates, relaxes, and revitalizes almost every part of your body. The Downward-Facing Dog is ideal for people who spend a lot of time sitting.

How:

1. Begin by kneeling on all fours with your hands directly under your shoulders and your knees directly under your hips. Move your hands forward about a palm's distance from their under-the-shoulder position (fig. 2-7a).

2. Inhale. Lift your hips up until you're standing on your toes. Keep the hands firmly planted on the floor and your legs straight. Your head, neck, arms, and back are all on an even plane (fig. 2-7b).

3. Exhale. With your weight evenly balanced,

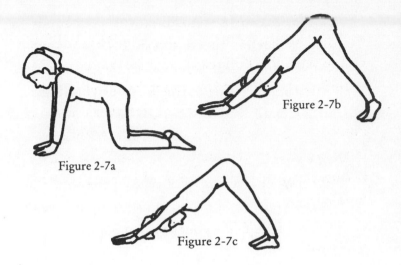

Figure 2-7a

Figure 2-7b

Figure 2-7c

drop your heels to the floor, feeling the
stretch in the Achilles tendons and calves.
Remain for a minimum of two breathing cycles (fig. 2-7c).
4. Return to a kneeling position.

Modifications:
* Instead of placing your hands on the floor,
  use the seat of a chair against a wall. This will
  lessen the intensity of the stretch consider-
  ably.

* At the close of the posture, with your hands and knees on the floor, sit back on your calves, drop your forehead to the floor, and stretch your arms out in front of you (Pose of a Child).

Remember:
* Keep your face and neck relaxed and soft.
* Keep your back, neck, and arms on an even plane. Don't lift your head up above your arms.
* Keep your weight evenly balanced between your feet and your hands. There is a tendency to allow the hands to carry most of the weight.
* This posture puts a lot of pressure on your wrists. If they are extremely sensitive, you may want to place a folded blanket underneath the heel of your palms, or avoid this posture altogether.

The Cobra

The long hours of forward bending, hunching,

and crunching that most of us do throughout the day cause our upper bodies to cry for a reverse stretch. The relief, flexibility, and strength that comes from a backward bending posture such as the Cobra is well worth the time it takes to learn it. This posture is good for rounded shoulders, and it also strengthens upper back muscles and the spine. Go slowly with the Cobra and remember that the movements don't have to be big to be effective. (People with disk problems should check with their doctor before doing this exercise.)

How:

1. Lie flat on your stomach, arms at your sides, legs together, your face looking down, your forehead resting on the floor (fig. 2-8a).
2. Inhale as you lift your hands up to either side of your shoulders and place your palms firmly on the floor. Your elbows are bent back. Your face is looking forward (fig. 2-8b).
3. Exhale as you brush your nose and then your chin across the floor, lifting your face until it is looking forward. Then, press your

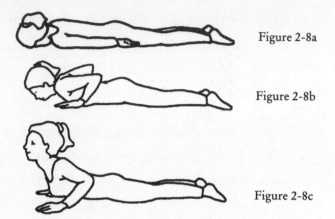

Figure 2-8a

Figure 2-8b

Figure 2-8c

hands into the floor and roll your upper back up a few inches, one vertebra at a time. Your eyes should look upward, your head gently tilted back. Don't lift your waist off the floor, only the upper back (fig. 2-8c).

4. Hold the position for at least one breathing cycle, then slowly roll back down, one vertebra at a time. Arms return to the sides, your forehead on the floor. Repeat.

Modifications:

* Instead of pressing your hands into the floor, try keeping your arms straight behind you and lifting your back in the same manner.

Keep your eyes facing forward (fig. 2-8d).

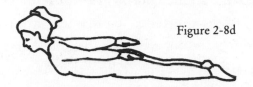

Figure 2-8d

Remember:

* Don't overbend. This posture is meant to stretch the upper back, not the lower back. Keep your naval flat on the floor.
* Use your arms to lift your body, not your neck. Keep the neck and throat relaxed.
* Keep your head from sinking into your shoulders. The shoulders shouldn't be compressed into the neck.
* Take it slow with this posture. Let your body adjust to it.

The Supine Hamstring Stretch

Most people have tight hamstrings. Runners and other athletes develop particularly tight hamstrings because of the repeated muscle contractions that occur in the back of the legs while running or jogging. Surprisingly, people who sit at a desk all day have a similar problem because their muscles adjust to the shortened, contracted sitting posture. Stretching the inherently inflexible hamstrings is necessary because the tighter they are, the greater the possibility for back, hip, and knee injuries. The Supine Hamstring Stretch is a simple, practical posture that gently lengthens your hamstrings without straining your lower back.

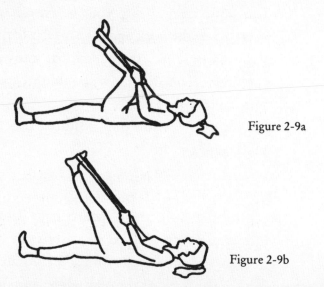

Figure 2-9a

Figure 2-9b

How:

1. Lie flat on your back with your legs straight.
2. Inhale. Bend your left leg and lift it up off the floor (fig. 2-9a). If your back is weak, keep the right leg bent with the right foot firmly planted on the floor.
3. Exhale. Wrap a belt or strap around your left foot and use both hands to pull the foot up as you straighten your left leg, continuing to lift it as high as possible. Press through your heel, not your toes (fig. 2-9b).
4. Hold the leg up as straight as possible for at least one breathing cycle and then slowly lower it. Perform an identical movement with the right leg.

Modifications:

* If you're limber, eliminate the belt and grab the toes of your left foot with your left hand. Push the foot up, keeping the leg straight and strong.

The Floor Twist

Twists relieve backaches, stiffness, headaches, and fatigue. They are wonderful to do after a long day of sitting in a car or at a desk. Twists can be done sitting, standing, or lying on the floor. They help the spine and hips remain supple and realign internal organs. The basic Floor Twist is just one of the many forms you can practice. If you have disk problems, check with your doctor before doing twists.

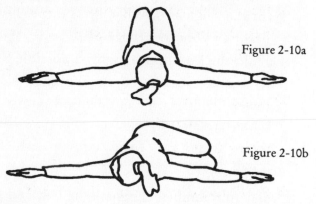

Figure 2-10a

Figure 2-10b

How:

1. Lay flat on your back, arms out to the sides at 90-degree angles to your body, palms flat on the floor, legs straight.

2. Inhale. Bring both knees into the chest. Your feet remain relaxed, calves parallel to the floor (fig. 2-10a).

3. Exhale. Roll your legs over to the left, keeping your right shoulder on the floor as much as possible and your knees bent. Your arms remain flat on the floor. Turn your head to the right, opposite of the direction you're rolling (fig. 2-10b).

4. Hold the pose for at least two breathing cycles, then roll back to the center and over to the right.

Modifications:

* Cross your right leg over your left before rolling to the left. This is known as the Secretary Twist.

* If you want to intensify the stretch as you turn to the left, rest your left hand on your right thigh and pull gently. To intensify the stretch as you turn to the right, rest your right hand on your left thigh and pull gently.

Remember:

* Let gravity pull your legs down. Don't force the stretch.
* Keep your arms flat.
* Turn your head away from the direction you're rolling.
* Be patient. You'll grow into this stretch. The more you do it, the better it feels.

The Pose of a Child

The Pose of a Child is good for relaxing and releasing your yoga experience. (For details on release work, refer to page 42, Release the Experience.) This comforting floor posture rests your back and legs. Note that there are a variety of options you can try if your body doesn't easily fold into the basic posture. If you find this pose too difficult, do the Corpse instead.

Figure 2-11

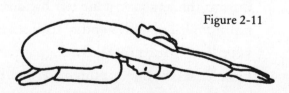

How:

1. Inhale. With your hands and knees on the floor, sit back on your calves, your hands resting on your knees.
2. Exhale. Bend over at the hips, stretching your arms out in front of you, your palms on the floor. Let your thighs support the weight of your torso. Relax into the pose with your forehead resting gently on the floor (fig. 2-11).
3. Hold the position for as long as is comfortable, releasing and relaxing. Acknowledge your efforts.
4. Inhale as you return to the starting position.

Modifications:

* If your thighs are tight, slip a towel or blanket between your thighs and calves.
* If your ankles and feet are tight, place a couple of folded blankets under your shins, with your feet hanging off the edge.
* Place a pillow under your forehead if your head doesn't reach the floor.

* Let your arms rest by your sides instead of stretching them out in front of you.

Remember:
* Keep breathing naturally and easily.
* Keep your toes pointed with the tops of your feet against the floor.
* Remain in the posture only as long as it is comfortable.

What would you think about a farmer who runs into his field one afternoon, throws corn seeds on the ground, dumps a season's worth of fertilizer and water on top of them, and is disappointed the next day when he doesn't see healthy, mature corn stalks? You'd think he was unrealistic, impractical, downright silly.

Yoga students often approach posture sequences with the same unrealistic expectations. In an effort to get the most out of the practice, they overextend through every posture and then give up in disgust when they don't see immediate change.

Immediacy has become our master in today's busy world. The need for instantaneous results has deadened our appreciation of the natural relationship between time and effort. In this relationship, the long-term picture must remain paramount or small efforts will be devalued and minor setbacks will cause despair.

As you do your posture sequences, try not to get bogged down by counting the day-to-day millimeters of change. Instead, look at yoga from a distance. See it as an ongoing process of ever-expanding health, ease, and awareness. Whether or not you bend a little farther today or tomorrow is of little consequence. What counts is that you keep practicing. To paraphrase an old Chinese maxim: It doesn't matter how slowly you go as long as you don't stop.

3

Practical Use

As you've probably already discovered, yoga is much more than just exercise — it's a holistic program that generates a relaxed equilibrium in your physical, mental, and emotional states. This equilibrium is immensely "practical" because it enables you to approach any event with clarity and responsive attention.

Yoga's sensible approach and philosophy reaches into every aspect of life. It helps counteract the physical and mental fatigue generated at the office. It establishes an emotional steadiness that helps you navigate through relationship anxiety. Yoga is especially suited to the rigors of travel, helping your body adjust to the many changes it must endure. Yoga also empowers you with the strength of emotional and physical authority.

The bad news is that you may not have time to do a full yoga sequence when you most need it. The good news is that yoga isn't limited to a rigidly defined sequence of postures. Yoga can fit into any time frame — a little bit of yoga goes a long way.

Yoga Bits and Their Applications

A yoga "bit" is a quick one-minute (or less) physical and mental refresher that can easily slip into your schedule. It consists of a single yoga posture, part of a posture, or a simple stretch that applies the principles of yoga. For example, if you work at a desk most of the time, you can use yoga bits throughout the day to revitalize your energy and alternately stimulate and stretch your legs and back. Yoga bits are appropriate under any circumstances and can be modified to fit any physical constraints. Yoga bits work in the car, at your desk, on a long plane flight, in a bus, standing in a grocery-store line, anywhere.

Combining yoga bits with regular yoga practice develops a sympathetic identification with your body. You learn to speak your body's language. You experience how a relaxed body supports a graceful mental state, and vice versa. Perhaps for the first time in your life, your body becomes your friend.

Yoga bits have two elements: the movement and the mind set. The first element, the movement, is the musculoskeletal lengthening, opening, and releasing of body tension. This relieves body fatigue and helps prevent long-term strain. The second element, the mind set, turns a static stretch into a mental refresher. The mind set helps relieve the annoying anxiety that often accompanies a busy schedule. It also enhances and deepens the effectiveness of the movement.

The Movement

The movement is simple. Take a portion of a yoga

posture and gently extend into it. It might be the overhead stretch from Step 1 of the Sun Salutation, or the Neck Stretches and Shoulder Rolls from the beginning of the standing sequence, or the sample yoga bits described later in this chapter.

Let's say you've been sitting at a desk for two or three hours. Your spine is compressed, your chest is sunken, and your body forms the shape of the letter C. Following the BS, BT reminder (page 51), begin your yoga bit by breathing deeply and smiling into a relaxed but alert condition. This first deep breath initiates a chest expansion which automatically breaks the unhealthy C shape. Going from bottom to top, place your feet squarely on the floor, making sure your weight is evenly distributed on your sitting bones. Pull your stomach in slightly to support the lower back and keep it from swaying. Scanning up the body, hang your arms loosely at your sides and do your first yoga bit — a nice, slow Shoulder Roll ending with the shoulders dropped into a relaxed position, the chest open, the collarbones broad. Keep your chin level, lift up from the top of your head and feel your back and neck elongate slightly, balancing the body in a seated position.

When you've aligned bottom-to-top (and of course while remembering to breathe), center your attention on one or two breathing cycles. (Refer to page 37, Center Your Attention.) You may decide to do a few more yoga bits, such as the Chest Opener and the Wall Rest. As you move from one yoga bit to the next, stay centered on what you're doing. Don't move your body without listening to it.

It takes longer to read the above description than to do it. You can condense the movement to a quick minute, even a matter of seconds, once you're used to performing yoga bits and you know the end result you're looking for.

The Mind Set

While the movement happens, your mind attends to the needs of your body. As you notice areas of tension, gently shift to relax those areas. Be mindful of your body's messages. Use the BS, BT reminder to deepen your breathing, relax your mouth and throat, and keep it light with a smile. Ah, it feels so good.

If you discover spots that are particularly knotted or sore, use a mental process to support the body work. Visualize the muscles and tendons relaxing, releasing into the movement. To assist you in this visualization, inhale deeply through your nose and imagine exhaling soft, silky air into those tight spots, soothing them like a balm. This visualization will deepen the stretch and refresh your mental state.

The mind set also includes releasing the experience of the yoga bit. This is particularly important because you may not have time to do as many yoga bits as you'd like, and it's easy to berate yourself for not doing "enough." Try not to dwell on what you can't do; acknowledge yourself for what you can do. If you only have time for one quick yoga bit, then do it, release it, and move on. You'll find that as you begin fitting yoga bits into your schedule, you'll naturally slide them in more frequently and with better results.

You may wonder how you can possibly

remember to do a yoga bit with a mind already saturated with shoulds and have-to's. Fortunately, there's a simple device you can use to help you establish the yoga bit habit — a cooking timer.

Set a cooking timer next to your desk or keep one in your car. If you have a computer, you might try using the system alarm clock. Set your timer every thirty to sixty minutes and train yourself to take a one-minute yoga break when the timer beeps. Before long, you'll develop a sensitive instinct that doesn't require an alarm to wake it up. You'll be able to give your mind and body quick refreshers whenever the need is apparent and return to the task at hand without missing a beat. Congratulations! You've fit yoga into your busy schedule!

YBP's Sample Yoga Bits

Just as there are countless posture sequence variations, there is also an unending variety of yoga bits that you can modify to suit your body's flexibility and skill level. The Shoulder Rolls and Neck Stretches from Chapter 2 are especially easy to do on the spur of the moment. As the principles of healthy movement become a natural part of your mind and behavior, you'll find yourself inventing all kinds of new yoga bits. You'll be sensitized to your body's subtle needs before they become problematic and you'll respond on the spot, creatively and effectively.

The yoga bits described in this chapter are basic; use this guide as an introduction to them. The order of execution (using YBP's three simple steps) is as follows: 1) center your attention with a deep breath; 2) perform the yoga bit; and 3) release the experience. Use the BS, BT reminder to relax and attend to your body's messages, movements, and the natural flow of your breathing.

Wrist Tendon-Easers

Wrist tendonitis is a common problem for people who do repetitive hand and wrist movements. Untreated, it can pave the way for more serious problems such as carpal tunnel syndrome. Fortunately, yoga is an excellent way to help prevent and manage wrist tendonitis. If you have recurring wrist problems, see your doctor and research wrist-strengthening yoga postures such as the Downward-Facing Dog. A word of caution — be very gentle with your wrists. Overstretching can make them worse, not better.

The Wrist Stretch

To ease the everyday strain from repetitive wrist movements, try the Wrist Stretch and the Palm Stretch below. The Wrist Stretch lengthens the muscles and tendons in the wrist, helping to reduce tension created from small, repetitive move-

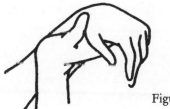

Figure 3-1

ments. It also stimulates blood flow to the area and increases the flexibility of the wrist.

How:

1. Place your right elbow on a desk or table with your right palm toward your face.
2. Let the weight of your left arm rest in the fingers of your right hand, gently stretching the right wrist backward (fig. 3-1). If you do this with your elbow on a table, let gravity stretch the wrist, assisted by the weight of your left arm. Hold for two to four breathing cycles, or up to thirty seconds.
3. When finished, gently bend the wrist forward to counteract the back bend. Repeat with the opposite wrist.

Modifications:

* If this stretch is too intense or you can't rest your arm anywhere, then simply pull the fingers gently back as far as feels comfortable.

Remember:

* You need to be fairly consistent with this stretch to begin to reverse the effects of tendonitis. Try to stretch your wrists at least once every thirty to sixty minutes.

* Be patient with your wrists. Don't over-stretch them in an effort to hasten the healing process.

The Palm Stretch

The Palm Stretch opens up the wrist by stretching out the palm and thumb. In conjunction with the Wrist Stretch, the Palm Stretch relieves stress in

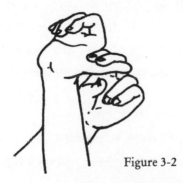

Figure 3-2

the hand and increases the overall flexibility of the wrist.

How:

1. Place your right elbow on a desk or table

with your right palm toward your face.

2. Bend the right wrist back by letting your left hand "hang" from your right thumb (fig. 3-2). Hold for two to four breathing cycles, or up to thirty seconds.

3. When finished, gently bend the wrist forward to counteract the back bend. Repeat with the opposite wrist.

Upper Body Relief

A busy person's stress frequently becomes trapped in the upper back between the shoulder blades, and in the muscles up the neck. This tension seeps into adjacent muscles in the chest and constricts the flow of breath. The Chest Opener can help release tension buildup before it becomes a problem.

The Chest Opener

The Chest Opener is a quick refresher that facilitates deep breathing and has a variety of forms. If you're not used to stretching in this manner, you

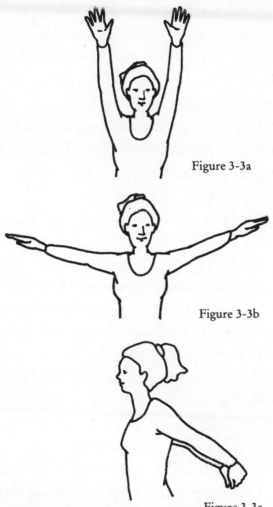

Figure 3-3a

Figure 3-3b

Figure 3-3c

may find it somewhat challenging at first, but the more you do it, the more you'll want to do it.

How:

1. Standing or sitting, stretch your arms straight up over your head, fingers outstretched but relaxed. Feel your body elongate as you reach up (fig. 3-3a). Hold for one or two deep breathing cycles.

2. Your arms remain straight as you begin to trace a large circle with your hands, moving them in opposite directions away from your body and down (fig. 3-3b). Slowly lower your arms until they are back down at your sides. Keep the shoulders soft and broaden the chest as you trace.

3. Seated or standing, with your arms behind your back and your sternum (breastbone) lifted, interlace your fingers and gently lift your arms back, keeping them as straight as you can (fig. 3-3c). If you find it difficult to lift your arms, then simply rest them behind your back with the fingers interlaced. Hold

for two breathing cycles.
4. Let your arms relax at your sides. Then repeat the same exercise two more times.

Modifications:

* After relaxing your arms at your sides, hug
  yourself across your chest to open the shoulder blades. Increase the stretch by letting
  gravity pull your chin down to your collarbone.

* If you're standing, find an open doorway,
  hang onto the sides of the door frame, and
  walk through the door until you feel a gentle
  stretch. You can move your arms up and

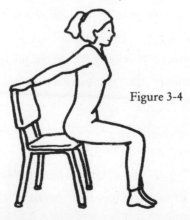

Figure 3-4

down the door frame to change the intensity and location of the stretch.

* If you're sitting, hook your arms behind the chair and lean slightly forward (fig. 3-4).
* If you have a friendly office mate, ask him or her to pull your arms back for you, so that you can completely relax into the stretch.

Remember:

* If you're standing, don't lock your knees. Keep your tailbone down. This prevents a sway back.
* Keep your shoulders down and your neck muscles soft. Don't strain.
* Keep the sternum lifted. Don't cave in your chest.
* If you feel like you're only stretching your arms, try the open doorway modification.

Lower Back Relief

You may have heard the saying that a chain will snap at its weakest link. For many busy people, the weak link is the lower back. Months of stress and a combination of weak stomach muscles, tight hamstrings, and hours of improper sitting or lifting can take a heavy toll. If you experience recurrent lower back trouble, consider committing to a combined program of back, leg, and stomach strengthening and stretching (yoga). It can make an enormous difference in your everyday comfort and mobility.

The Wall Rest

The Wall Rest helps combat nagging lower back discomfort. If you sit at a desk all day, the

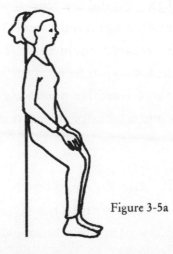

Figure 3-5a

Wall Rest counteracts exhaustion produced by a rounded spine. If you stand on your feet all day, the Wall Rest takes the burden from your lower back and gives your legs a break by using the wall to help support you.

How:

1. Stand with your back to a wall, feet shoulder-width apart, twelve inches from the floorboard.

2. Press your back against the wall and lengthen your spine so that your lower back rests flat. Imagine that every part of your back is pressed against the wall. Bend your knees as necessary to achieve a flat back, but be sure to keep your knees over your ankles (fig. 3-5a). Remain in this pose as long as you're comfortable, or progress into the Wall Squat.

Remember:

* Breathe abdominally to increase the restful nature of this stretch.

* Keep your knees from extending forward, in

front of the ankles, or locking into a straight line from ankle to hip.

The Wall Squat

The Wall Squat is an effective stretch for the lower back and the Achilles tendons in the backs of the ankles. It also strengthens the lower legs. Unfortunately, most people's Achilles tendons are too tight to allow them to settle into a proper heels-on-the-floor squat. The Wall Squat circumvents this problem by using the wall to support the back and maintain proper balance. As you slide down the wall, your heels remain planted on the floor and your Achilles tendons get a good, healthy stretch. A word of caution: If your knees

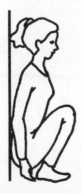

Figure 3-5b

are sensitive or injured, check with your doctor before attempting a Wall Squat.

How:
1. Do the Wall Rest.
2. Slide your flattened back down toward the floor until you are in a squat position. You may need to adjust your feet somewhat, but they should still be flat on the floor (fig. 3-5b). Pushing your elbows against the wall keeps you balanced in this posture.
3. To finish the posture, either slide your feet forward until you're sitting on the floor, or simply roll over to the side and stand up.

Modifications:
* Open a door and hang onto the door knobs as you squat.
* Face a partner and grasp your partner's wrists as both of you squat down simultaneously. The pull from your partner will counterbalance your tendency to fall backward.

Remember:

* If your knees hurt, stop.
* Keep your heels on the floor.
* Don't overtax your knees and legs the first time you do this. Gradually increase the time you spend in the stretch.

The Standing Chair Hang

The Standing Chair Hang is a quick and easy way to stretch your lower back after a long day sitting at your desk. Its value is enhanced when followed by the Sitting Chair Hang.

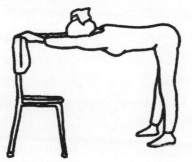

Figure 3-6

How:

1. Stand about three feet behind a stable chair. Grab the back of a chair with your hands,

placing them about twelve inches apart.

2. Keeping your arms and legs straight, bend forward at the hips, letting the trunk of your body lengthen down between your arms. Your hips and thighs should be moving away from your hands (fig. 3-6). Relax for at least three breathing cycles.

3. To finish the posture, step toward the chair, release the chair back, and slowly roll up, one vertebra at a time. If you like, do it again from a seated position.

Modifications:

* If your lower back is stronger, stand up straight and bend over at the hips, keeping your arms, upper body, and head hanging loose. Keep your knees strong but unlocked. Let gravity do the work. Relax for at least three breathing cycles. Then bend your knees and slowly roll up one vertebra at a time.

Remember:

* The transition from hanging to standing tall

must occur gently. A slow upward roll gives an extra stretch to your spine and prevents possible dizziness.

The Sitting Chair Hang

Create a simple, effective yoga break for your back and your mind with the Sitting Chair Hang.

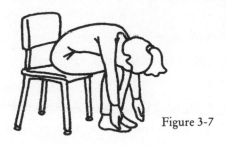

Figure 3-7

How:

1. Sit comfortably in a chair with your legs together, your feet flat on the floor.
2. With your weight evenly distributed on your sitting bones, rest your upper body in your lap as you let your arms hang down by your legs (fig. 3-7). Relax for at least three breathing cycles.

3. To finish the posture, place your hands on your knees and use your arms to help you roll up, one vertebra at a time.

Modifications:

* Bring the arms forward after letting them hang straight down. This increases the stretch to the back.

Remember:

* Because this pose compresses the abdomen as you bend forward, you may find it difficult to take deep abdominal breaths. Just breathe as naturally and easily as you can.
* As with the Standing Chair Hang, the transition from resting in your lap into an upright seated position must occur gently. A slow upward roll gives an extra stretch to your spine and prevents possible dizziness.

Leg Stretches

Many back problems find their source not in

the back, but in the legs. Tight hamstrings pull on the lower back. As the leg muscles lose their elasticity and strength, they also leave you vulnerable to knee and hip injuries. Fortunately, many problems can be avoided with regular practice of the Ham Stretch. If you have time, perform the Warrior before the Ham Stretch to maximize the lengthening of the hamstrings.

The Ham Stretch

The Ham Stretch can be done anywhere, using a chair, a table, even the stairs. Because the hamstrings are stubborn and inflexible, you should do

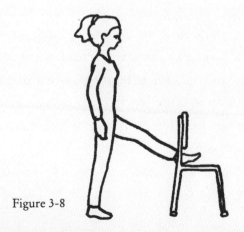

Figure 3-8

this yoga bit more than once a day. Fit it in while talking on the phone, waiting for an appointment, or on a break between meetings.

How:

1. Stand about two feet away from a chair or table. Make sure your weight is evenly balanced over both feet.

2. Facing the chair, place your left foot on the seat, straightening your left leg. Relax your left foot and extend out through the heel (fig. 3-8).

3. If you don't feel a stretch up the back of your left leg, lean forward at the hips until you do. Rest your hands gently on your leg as you lean forward. Hold the stretch (no bouncing!) for at least two breathing cycles.

4. Remove your leg from the chair, relax for a moment, and then repeat the same stretch over again.

5. Repeat the same movements with the right leg.

Modifications:

* As you become more flexible, increase the height of the chair or table.
* Stand sideways next to the chair, lift your leg onto the chair and, with your hands on your hips, bend sideways over your leg. The toes and the knee of the uplifted leg should face the ceiling.

Remember:

* Your elevated leg should be in front of your body, not to the side. This isn't a side bend.
* If you have to lean forward too far, your foot isn't high enough. Find a taller chair or use a table.
* As you bend forward, visualize extending your head out toward your toes. This helps the back to remain long.
* Try to keep your knees strong but unlocked.

Using Yoga Bits in a Variety of Settings

The calmness, clarity, and focus of yoga combines to create a powerful stabilizing influence, useful in a variety of everyday settings. As you proceed through the responsibilities of your day — working at the office, dealing with family and relationships, even traveling — yoga bits revive the sensory memory (and reward) of the yoga sequence itself.

Office Yoga

As the conduit for our financial security and (often) the center of our anxieties, work takes on great importance in our lives. We spend more time working than we spend doing anything else. For most of us, this means little exercise and a lot of sitting. Even physically demanding jobs tend to be centered around repetitive movements, overextending some muscles and leaving others untouched. Modern day work doesn't usually harmonize with the body; it unbalances it.

The problems of work are more than just

physical. A sour combination of frustration and competition can cook into a stew of anxiety. This emotional ragout simmers for days until, one morning, you bend over to tie your shoe and the weight of it pours into your lumbar spine, sending you to the back specialist. Or you develop a nagging knot under your shoulder blade. Or, for so many computer users today, the tendons in your wrists inflame.

Many busy people value these disorders as the proud backwash of success. But body pain and its psychological counterpart, anxiety, is debilitating. It dulls your senses and ages you mentally and physically. It also weakens you, making you susceptible to illness and even injury.

Fortunately for all of us, a little bit of yoga in the workplace can help reverse this unhealthy trend. For example, here's how I use yoga bits while I work.

Like many people, I'm glued to a desk much of the day. So every hour or so, I do a yoga bit. It may be a three-posture sequence next to my desk, or a quick tendon-easer. I initially had to set a timer to force the breaks in my schedule, but they made such a difference in my overall health and well-being that they quickly became habitual. These breaks usually include a variety of Chest Openers (figs. 3-3 a–c) to counteract the hunching and tension in my shoulders. They also include deep, abdominal breathing. Deep breathing lowers the anxiety that may be building if I'm under deadline pressure, and also wakes me up if I'm getting a little groggy.

John, a busy college instructor, has also successfully incorporated yoga bits into the workplace. John used to suffer from leg pain and lower back problems due to long hours of standing on his feet. "I was having a lot of trouble with my back," John explains. "But after a week of doing little stretches during the day, I noticed a difference in my back and also in my mind. I just wasn't as tense."

The yoga bits John uses are simple. They include Wall Rests to relax his back, deep breathing to minimize the tiredness that comes from lecturing, and Ham Stretches and Wall Squats during breaks between classes. He also performs Neck Stretches and Shoulder Rolls throughout his work day, visualizing the muscles loosening and relaxing. "It sounds like a lot of time," John says, "but it really takes only a minute or so. I'm amazed at how much better I feel at the end of the day. Yoga really works."

John feels better because he's doing more than just stretching on occasion. He's invested in the mind and body benefits he receives from the practice. He fits it in whenever he can and his results speak for themselves. "I can't imagine how I ever got along without it," he says.

Relationship Yoga

Next to work stress, relationship stress is probably the most tiresome issue busy people encounter. And even though yoga won't necessarily change your relationships, regular practice will build up a savings of emotional equilibrium that can serve you well if the going gets rough.

Most of us don't emotionally detonate at the drop of a hat. There's usually significant buildup.

A bad day at the office makes us defensive. A stressful drive on the freeway adds to our frustrations. By the time we get home, we're ready to do battle over the smallest annoyance.

Yoga bits counteract this emotional buildup because they reduce tension. Yoga helps calm the body and gives the mind enough of a focus to keep it from obsessing and overreacting. It's difficult for the mind to remain upset when the muscles are quiet and the breathing is deep.

Let's say you're about to discuss a particularly sensitive subject with your partner. You can feel yourself becoming anxious because you know the subject matter generates conflict. The moment you become aware of the anxiety, immediately begin diffusing it with yoga bits. Try to do a stretch that relaxes the area of your body most affected by your mental state. For example, if you want to shout, do Neck Stretches and deep breathing. If you're burdened by negligence, try stretching your back or rolling your shoulders to shrug off the anxiety. If you feel weak, insecure, or unworthy, then stand tall and balanced, breathe deeply, and do a bottom-to-top alignment scan to connect yourself to your own sureness. If possible, these yoga bits should be performed before the discussion occurs; however, because they take only seconds, they can be slipped in whenever you need them. Remember that as you stretch, take a deep breath and center your attention. This helps establish clear thinking.

Yoga won't fundamentally change your feelings or dispel your passion. However, it will help you to function more effectively through those feelings. You may hear an angry voice inside your head, but your emotional equilibrium will give you the freedom to not act on its message.

I'm not saying that a little bit of yoga here and there will solve all your problems. Yoga isn't a magic bullet. But it does increase your awareness so you are less likely to respond inappropriately. Consistent yoga practice helps to keep you emotionally buoyant and level-headed. You begin to see alternatives and new directions. The lens through which you view life expands, because you're not as rigid and guarded. And it helps you stay healthy, too.

Travel Yoga

If there's one thing a busy person needs to learn, it's how to travel with minimal stress. Whether it's the daily commute to work, a trip across country to visit relatives, or a business trip lasting several days, travel is necessary and sometimes arduous. Physical constraints in planes, trains, and cars constrict the muscles in your back and neck. Legs quickly become fatigued as they're forced into cramped positions with little room for movement. The mental and emotional agitation that often accompanies travel can be equally tiresome.

Travel contains three major stressors: 1) the physical stress of sitting for long periods of time in planes, cars, or buses; 2) the performance stress of attending business meetings and family get togethers; and 3) the schedule-related stress of tossing your familiar eating and exercising patterns out the window.

1. *Physical stress:* Physically, your body is built for movement; sitting for extended periods of time in cramped jets, cars, or buses is tedious and unnatural. Yoga bits are made-to-order for counteracting the negative effects of long-term sitting or standing. Try the Ham Stretch, the Wall Squat, the Neck Stretch, and the Floor Twist. Breathe soothing care into the tension, clearly instructing the muscles to relax and stay loose. A good, brisk walk is also helpful.

2. *Performance stress:* Most travel involves performing in a variety of ways. If it's a business trip, you're playing the role of knowledgeable professional. If it's a family gathering, you're being a loving child, successful sibling, or devoted spouse. If it's a vacation, you're being a relaxed, happy traveler. Perhaps your greatest challenge in life is to be as real and honest in each of these roles as you can possibly be.

The purpose of this book isn't to explore the many roles in life that you juggle; rather, it is to show you how yoga can help you function within those roles, despite the apprehension they sometimes generate. Whatever type of performance anxiety you're experiencing, a little bit of yoga can help you weather it effectively. For example, taking deep abdominal breaths will stop the shallow chest breathing that accompanies dread or concern — you'll think more clearly. Stretching into the Warrior will generate a sense of strength and authority — you'll feel more powerful. A little healthy exploration will teach you which postures work best.

3. *Schedule stress:* Whenever you travel for business or pleasure, you have to expect the unexpected. Maintaining a regular schedule of yoga is difficult. If you're too rigid, you'll become overanxious. If you're too lenient, you won't ever get around to doing it.

Many traveling yoga aficionados practice their

yoga first thing in the morning, right after showering. If you wait much longer, there's a good chance other issues will take priority. Also, keep your yoga sequences very short. If they're much longer than ten minutes, your mind can procrastinate with, "I just don't have the time right now. Maybe after lunch." Resolve to go through the day fitting in yoga bits here and there to help compensate for the stress. If you have time in the evening, do another sequence before retiring. If you don't have time, don't sweat it.

Everybody confronts obstacles at one time or another. It could be a relationship breakup, a financial problem, a health issue, or anything that triggers fear and a sense of powerlessness. Nowhere is the mind/body connection more apparent: As emotions ignite, the body tightens. As anxiety surfaces, the breath shortens.

When you feel powerless, you unconsciously look for ways to regain your sense of authority. Strong emotion is often a product of powerlessness because it fuels the body with a rush of adrenaline. Unfortunately, this power is capricious. It relies on drama to pump itself up, and it fluctuates with the ups and downs of your moods.

Yoga empowers you in the same way strong emotion does, but without the negative repercussions. Yoga balances your feelings so that the strength isn't chained to emotional caprice and hormonal rushes. Your strength is resilient, proactive, and poised. Your thinking remains unobstructed and there's room for a solution orientation.

Prove it to yourself. As you begin practicing yoga, using yoga bits throughout the day, watch your point of view change. Observe your options increase as your mind relaxes and your spine lengthens. When you experience a challenge in your life, take a break and do some yoga. Feel your horizons expand. Feel your alternatives emerge. It's glorious.

4

Staying Motivated

B usy people are often so inundated with responsibilities that they feel unable to invest much energy into maintaining new, unfamiliar practices such as yoga. They often "run on empty," barely getting through the daily demands already placed on them by work and family. Busy folks may eagerly start a yoga program, but later give it up, succumbing to frustration and loss of interest. The problem is that most people don't know how to maintain enough motivation to endure through the initial decline in enthusiasm. Once they lose the sizzle, they lose their drive.

Fortunately, motivation is something that can be encouraged and augmented. In this chapter you'll learn about a variety of creative and interesting ways to reawaken your motivation. These simple suggestions can help you triumph over old habits, keep you moving forward, and give you the edge you need to succeed.

How to Keep Yourself Motivated

When you're enthusiastic, you're also motivated; however, you can also be motivated but not particularly enthusiastic. For example, many cardiac patients are strongly motivated to change their lifestyles, but they are seldom enthusiastic about it. The physical threat of illness is their change agent, not the joy of living without saturated fat.

Enthusiasm is delightful, but it's only one kind of motivation. In fact, motivation is divided into three parts: emotional, intellectual, and physical. Seldom are all three equally proportioned. While emotional motivation (a.k.a. enthusiasm) is the most familiar, often it's physical and intellectual motivation that provide the sturdiest foundation for change.

Get Enthusiastic!

If you've ever heard a stirring speech, you know what emotional motivation feels like. It's a passionate charge that promotes immediate action and makes your dreams seem within reach. If you think of your life as a horse race, emotional motivation is what breaks you out of the gate. That burst of enthusiasm gets your hooves pounding down the track.

Emotional motivation isn't supposed to be a sustained experience; it's a peak, a high. Enthusiastic peaks are separated by plateaus of energy and effort. Fortunately, you have some control over how wide your plateaus are. By learning how to get out of your head and into your heart, you can actually shorten the distance between peaks.

Enthusiasm is a heartfelt experience. To effectively generate it, you have to take a lesson from children — learn how to play. When you play, your emotions are set free and creativity is unleashed. Options expand and you become eager again. If you find yourself falling into the old habit of ignoring yoga in favor of endless business meetings or other mundane responsibilities, it's probably time to regenerate your enthusiasm. And what better way to get enthusiastic than to play! Try playing around with a few of these ideas:

1. *Vary your sequence order or add new postures.* Adding new postures will enliven regular practice. Just remember that you must season newness with maturity. Don't throw away what's tried and true (and what works for you) simply for the sake of variety. Continue to spend time in the more familiar poses, even as you add new ones. Yoga postures are friends. As the old chestnut goes, "Make new friends but keep the old. One is silver and the other is gold."

2. *Create a yoga corner.* Carving out a symbolic niche, even if it's only the corner of a room, reinforces commitment. It makes your practice an undeniable part of your life. At home, your

yoga corner can include a table for your props, maybe a small bookcase, even a few encouraging photos. One student put a big stop sign in her yoga space, reminding her to stop and do it. At the office you probably need to be more subtle. Try hanging a yoga calendar on the wall opposite your desk.

3. *Wear a yoga outfit that makes you feel good.* A special outfit helps separate practice time from the rest of your schedule. When you change from work clothes into a sweat suit or even a loose shirt reserved especially for yoga, you symbolically shed the anxieties of the day. You begin to settle down, even before your first posture.

4. *Explore interesting and unusual props.* Research into yoga will reveal a variety of props you can use to help achieve proper alignment in postures. Use chairs, doorways, belts, blocks, pillows — anything that adds dimension to your practice. Care must be taken with props. They're a waste of time if they aren't helping

you relax deeply into your pose or maintain proper alignment. To avoid dependency, vary their inclusion into your sequence. After all, it might be awkward to say to your boss, "I'd like to do a quick hamstring stretch. Could I borrow your belt?"

5. *Use music to accompany your practice.* On occasion I've used Gregorian chants, various symphonies, even sounds of the rain forest. Unfortunately, music does have a couple of drawbacks: It can seduce attention away from the yoga posture itself, and it encourages dependency. To avoid these problems, try to keep your musical selections low key, and don't play music every time you do yoga. Make your music a special treat.

6. *Find a yoga buddy.* Human beings are social creatures; we learn more quickly and thoroughly through interactions with other people. If you can arrange to do your yoga with a friend at least once a week, you're not only more likely to continue practicing, you'll also enjoy it more.

Get Smart!

Good trainers and seminar leaders don't count on emotions to keep their workshop participants productive. They know that when emotional investment wanes, something else has to keep their students involved. That something is often the reasoning mind, bolstered by useful information, stimulating ideas, and practical techniques. Intellectual motivation carries you from one oasis of enthusiasm to the next. When properly equipped, your intellect can literally argue you into an activity you would otherwise avoid. Here are some ways to trigger intellectual motivation:

1. *Do a reality check.* Yoga practice loses its priority when you stop noticing how good you feel. After a few weeks, the limber joints, the relaxed back, the general feeling of well-being become commonplace. Your perspective changes and you start to forget why yoga was so important to you. A single-sentence reality check can help jog your memory:

"Before I started yoga, my body and mind felt _____; since I took up yoga, my body and mind feel _____. What a difference!"

If you want to motivate yourself, then your reality check must be spoken aloud and with gusto. Shout it in your car. Call friends on the phone and tell them. Announce it to the mirror. Say it until your intellect finally pushes through your amnesia.

2. *Study yoga.* Yoga is a well-documented subject. Reading about yoga and its life-enhancing properties is as fascinating as it is inspiring. Libraries are full of books and videos on the topic. Appendix 1 lists a few favorites.

3. *Prioritize your practice.* How important is it to stretch, strengthen, and rebuild your body? How necessary is it to detox from daily pressure and anxiety? How badly do you need physical and emotional relaxation? When you prioritize yoga as urgent and important, you commit yourself to doing it. Sincere commitment helps push through habitual procrastination and

avoidance behavior.

4. *Tell yourself it's more than just exercise.* If you have a history of procrastinating with exercise, then remind yourself that yoga is much more than exercise. The positive repercussions of yoga flow into every aspect of your life. The strength helps you tolerate brutal body postures assumed during a standard work day. The flexibility helps prevent injuries and keeps you supple and youthful. The mind/body energy exchange supports a mental clarity and focus that makes you more efficient and more pleasant to be around. Who can argue with these benefits?

5. *Take a yoga class.* Yoga classes are wonderful. Yoga teachers are often storehouses of physiological and philosophical information. Learning yoga from someone who has been studying and practicing it for years is not only immensely practical, it's also utterly fascinating. The combination of teacher guidance, class support, and informative books is a potent prescription for keeping up practice.

6. *Use a calendar.* Mark each day you complete a yoga sequence. (Be very generous with yourself. If you do a single Sun Salutation, mark the day.) Research has shown that people who keep a record of their successes tend to continue being successful. Reviewing a calendar full of X's is satisfying and stimulating. It's also an excellent visual reminder.

Get Physical!

When I was in my mid-twenties, I held a high-stress management position. Being a young professional with a lot to prove, I didn't pay attention to the nagging sciatic pain in my legs or the growing knots in my neck. I didn't have the time or the inclination to attend to my body. Then one day, I got up from my desk and couldn't walk out of the office without assistance. My doctor prescribed four days of bed rest. If my back didn't improve in a week, I'd have to see an orthopedic surgeon.

It's not an unfamiliar story. Human beings have the remarkable power of selective attention. We can so effectively ignore the physically motivating messages that our bodies send us (messages such as *I need to stretch, I need to walk around, I need to relax*), that we actually become deaf to them. This selective attention may be a necessity if you're in a marathon race, but most of us don't ignore our bodies out of necessity. We do it out of convenience. It's difficult to find time to relax. It's inconvenient to stretch. We ignore our bodies' needs and then suffer the consequences of stress, chronic fatigue, and illness. One thing is certain: the body always has the final word.

The threat of surgery was a body message I chose not to ignore. It wasn't easy, but after months of yoga, physical therapy, and a few lifestyle changes, I eased back into a functional body. I learned a painful, expensive lesson. Now, when my body speaks to me, I make every effort to respond. I'm not perfect by any means, but I avoid a lot of problems, and I no longer have back trouble.

Yoga helps you learn how to hear your body's messages. Yoga is designed to sensitize you. After only a few sessions, you'll begin to hear not only your body's requests for movement, but you'll also feel how wonderful it is to respond to those requests. Does your neck need to lengthen after sinking into your shoulders all day? Do your hamstrings need to stretch after running up three flights of stairs to get to the office on time? When you let your body motivate you, you live a more robust life of vitality and youthful vigor.

If you don't know how to listen to your body's messages, take heart. Here are a few simple suggestions to get you going:

1. *Have a chat with your body.* Make friends with your body by learning how to talk with it. Ask your body what it needs and listen carefully to its responses. This is an excellent way to develop your inner ear — the ear that hears your body's motivating messages. For example, after teaching a three-hour seminar, I often take a quick break to ask my body what it needs from me. (I've learned not to assume that it will always need the same thing!) Sometimes it wants

to walk a few blocks. Sometimes it wants to do yoga. Sometimes it just wants to collapse in a big chair and eat something tasty.

2. *Associate everyday activities with body chats.* For example, if you get in and out of the car frequently during the day, associate opening the car door with a body chat. Every time you grab the car-door handle, stand still for a moment and ask your body what it needs. It may need you to take off your shoes for few minutes to relax your feet. It may need some rejuvenating deep breaths or a quick stretch. It may be fine as is. The point is that you're using familiar tasks to "cue" you to listen and respond to your body's messages.

3. *Use the golden-cord alignment practice.* The orientation of your head in relation to your neck and shoulders is a clear message about the condition of your upper body as well as your energy level. When you develop the habit of noticing the position of your head and neck, you'll be able to quickly correct potential alignment problems, ward off upper

body discomfort, and, as a result, increase your energy.

The golden-cord practice is a simple visualization that concentrates your attention on your body's alignment. First, imagine a golden cord pulling you straight up from the crown of your head. Next, observe your chin level. If your chin tilts up, the cord is pulling you backward. If your chin drops toward your chest, the cord is pulling you forward. In either case, you need to straighten the pull of your cord. This simple visualization will help you maintain a straight, aligned posture, regardless of your current activity.

4. *Use the back-of-head alignment practice.* When your posture is correct, it's much easier to hear your body's motivating messages. If you sit at a desk all day, your posture probably suffers from the neck down. The back-of-head alignment practice is a simple, useful visualization that can help you correct your posture and wake you up if you're feeling sleepy.

Notice the back of your head. If it's sinking into your shoulders, you're stressing your neck, shoulders and upper back, and you've probably lost focus on what you're doing. By lifting up from the crown of the head, you inject energy into your posture and your focus becomes realigned along with your body.

Keeping on Track

There are two methods commonly used to fit yoga into a busy schedule: the do-it-whenever method and the scheduled method. Both methods work — you just have to decide which works best for you.

The do-it-whenever method gives you a lot of space. "Whenever" is sometime during the course of a day. This method slips yoga into your schedule without making too many demands. It works if you're already fairly disciplined or if you have a yoga buddy living in the same house with you. The do-it-whenever method gives you room to maneuver and rebel.

The scheduling method is appropriate if you need less space and more structure. It also prevents your mind from obsessing about yoga whenever you have a break in the day. "Hmm, I should have done it this morning. Maybe I should do it now. No, I can fit it in after lunch. Maybe I should do it this evening. Maybe...." By the end of the day, your mind will feel like you've been doing yoga for hours, even though you haven't executed a single posture.

There are three questions to ask yourself before deciding whether or not to include yoga in a written schedule:

1) Are you worried about fitting yoga practice into your busy day?
2) Are you a chronic procrastinator?
3) Regardless of how enthusiastic you are about yoga, do you detect any resistance to doing it?

If you answer yes to at least two of these questions, you should probably use a schedule.

Scheduling is important to busy procrastinators because:

1. *It initiates action.* Writing something down moves it from fantasy to reality. When you schedule yoga, you're telling yourself it is serious. You're demonstrating resolve.

2. *It sustains commitment.* When you see yoga written on a weekly schedule, you've made a place for it in your life. You're more likely to keep up your practice.

3. *It relieves your mind.* What a relief to be able to say to yourself, "Oh, yoga is scheduled for 4:30." Period. No obsessing. No question. When yoga time rolls around, you'll be ready for it.

To use a schedule effectively, only include activities that you resist doing such as exercise, studying, going to the dentist, and so on. Packing your schedule with too many tasks could generate discouragement or rebellion. If you start to feel choked, then schedule in blocks of free time so you can say to yourself, "See? I do have time!"

Also, keep your schedule visible and flexible. Stick it on your refrigerator and write it in pencil. If things don't work out, erase them and change the date. Don't make a big production out of it. As a busy person you have to reschedule appointments all the time. It isn't a sign of failure, it's just another schedule change. What's important here is your intention. If you intend to find a way to fit yoga into your life, you'll succeed in doing so. You may hit some rough spots and resistance, but you'll succeed in the long run and the results will be well worth your efforts.

Combining Yoga with Other Exercise

If you're not currently involved with an exercise program, yoga should be where you start. If you already exercise, yoga will enhance the value of your current activity by elongating your muscles, helping your joints move freely, and offering a form of deep rejuvenation that most other types of exercise don't provide. If you're already an athlete, then yoga is an absolute must to prevent injuries and counteract the muscular imbalances that develop as a result of overuse and specialized training. No matter what form of exercise you do, yoga can make a big difference in your success with it.

Yoga is appropriate before and after any form of exercise. For example, if you're an aerobic dancer, you should do about ten minutes of yoga before and after your workout. The same is true for bicycling, running, even weight lifting. Before exercise, yoga prepares your body to absorb the stress of movement. It helps your muscles flex with the activity instead of tighten against it, thus helping to prevent injuries. It also steadies your mental state so that your workout is executed with attention and efficacy. Afterward, yoga helps balance the muscles that were over- or under-used during exercise. It neutralizes the muscles' tendency to contract and become inflexible. This muscle balancing is critical to the prevention of future injuries. Yoga also encourages the flushing of lactic acid, helping you recover from your workout more quickly and with less discomfort.

Going to Class

Yoga class is a motivational treat to give yourself. It's one of the surest ways to rekindle your enthusiasm. Even a few short classes can refine and revitalize your practice. Beyond the externally enforced discipline of regular attendance, there's perhaps the greatest class benefit — the instructor.

Picking a Good Instructor

At some point in your yoga experience, you'll probably want the input of another individual. A person who can look at you with compassionate dispassion and say, "That's very nice, but why don't we move your knee a little more like this," changing your entire experience of a posture. This person is your yoga instructor.

In North America, the influx of information and yoga teaching styles have created a dynamic hodgepodge of forms taught by instructors with vastly different backgrounds and agendas. But good instructors have certain similarities that transcend all stylistic differences. They are skilled teachers with ample room in their repertoire of postures for your physical limitations. They generate enthusiasm and belief in the minds of their students because they practice what they preach.

If you're considering taking a class, talk to students who've worked with the instructor in the past. How do they feel about the quality of instruction? Were they comfortable asking questions? Were they encouraged to read supplementary materials? Take some time also to talk directly to the instructor. Discuss any specific injuries you may have, such as weak knees or a sensitive back. (Some instructors specialize in back problems or structural abnormalities; others are general practitioners.) Ask if you can attend one session on a trial basis to see if the class is appropriate for you. And if everything feels good, get ready for a delightful experience.

Getting the Most Out of Class

Yoga class is an excellent investment in time

and energy, but the benefit you derive is in direct proportion to your willing participation. If you sign up for class and then don't go, you're wasting money and missing out on an enriching experience. If you go to class but avoid asking for help because you're too embarrassed or self-conscious, you're minimizing the value of the instruction. To receive the greatest benefit from class, follow these basic guidelines:

1. *Go when you don't feel like it.* The best time to do yoga is when you don't feel like doing it. Yoga isn't a practice only for the days when you feel limber. It's meant to work with your body regardless of its current condition. Yoga channels energy through the structure of the body, revitalizing you no matter how bad you feel.

2. *While you're in class, be in class.* Don't spend your posture time thinking about lunch, work, or anything else. This is a gift you've given yourself. A gift of time and attention. Don't cheat yourself with thoughts you can think just

as easily after class concludes.

3. *Make peace with imperfection.* A body that has been cramming itself into cars, office chairs, and improperly fitting shoes for years isn't going to flow easily into every posture. Fortunately, yoga is more than posture. In the classic sense, yoga is the physical path toward unifying the body, mind, and spirit. The "goal" isn't perfect posture. It's unity.

4. *Don't compare yourself to anyone else.* Comparisons are part of human nature. You can't help but indulge in them now and then. But you have to decide why you paid for the class in the first place. Is it to be the best you can be, or to do a backbend like a gymnast half your age? On the practical side, you might ask the instructor if there are classes specifically designed for your age group or skill level. Also, certain classes may attract different crowds depending on the time the class is held.

5. *Don't eat before class.* Never eat heavily before any exercise class. The activity can disturb your digestion and may make you uncomfortable.

6. *Don't give up.* The first few weeks can be emotionally as well as physically uncomfortable,
   particularly if you're less flexible than the rest
   of the class. Everyone is a little self-conscious.
   Just allow the embarrassment or general discomfort to sit alongside of you without giving
   it too much attention. Eventually, it will disin-
   tegrate, being replaced by the pleasure you receive from class.

Whenever you try to develop a new practice or
habit, it's like you're on a small boat navigating
through a reed-choked river. Boredom, frustration,
and procrastination ripple out from your boat as
you attempt to forge through tangles of distractions and responsibilities. The problem for many of
us is that we worry so much about the ripples, we
forget to properly steer the boat. If we see boredom
rippling through the water, we think that the new
route we're attempting no longer has value. If we
see frustration and procrastination, we assume that
the new route is unsuitable because it's challenging.
Try to remember, it's human nature to struggle

against change. Resistance doesn't always mean that what you resist is wrong for you. It usually means that your routines are being questioned and other alternatives are being explored. Charting a new course can sometimes generate a little rough water. If you stay motivated, persistent, and willing to ask for help when you need it, you'll push through the rushes, disregard the ripples, and discover a whole new passage to health and vitality.

Appendix 1

Reference Tools

You never learn all there is to know about yoga because as your mind opens and your boundaries expand, old information takes on new meaning.

Although *Yoga for Busy People* provides a good basis for starting your practice, it remains deliberately simple in many areas. The following books and videos are excellent for further study as well as for general reading. There are countless other fine works available.

Reading Material

The Runner's Yoga Book: A Balanced Approach to Fitness, Jean Couch (Berkeley, CA: Rodmell Press, 1990). An excellent guide to the intricate details of yoga postures. Written for athletes, it is also appropriate for beginners because of the exceptional photographic depictions of the various postures as well as Jean Couch's easy-to-understand prose and the exceptionally clear photographs.

Living Yoga, Georg Feuerstein & Stephen Bodian (Los Angeles: Jeremy P. Tarcher, Inc., 1993). An accessible, beautifully compiled series of *Yoga Journal's* finest essays, articles, interviews, and photographs.

Yoga, the Iyengar Way, Silva, Mira & Shyam Mehta (New York: Alfred A. Knopf, Inc., 1990). This book explains the basic principles and practices of yoga. Based on the authors' thirty years of study with B. K. S. Iyengar. Excellent photos and descriptive text.

Yoga Journal. A magazine dedicated to communicating the qualities of being that yoga exemplifies. Includes excellent articles on health, lifestyle, and contemporary applications of Hatha yoga. It also publishes exquisite calendars. Well-researched, stimulating, very readable. Everyone should subscribe to it.

Yoga International. A magazine with a distinctly holistic, spiritual mission. Includes articles on body/mind/spirit integration, meditation, yoga, and vegetarian eating. Also includes interviews with respected spiritual teachers and seekers.

Vegetarian Times. A magazine that educates and supports a vegetarian lifestyle. Often includes articles on stress reduction, health issues, and yoga. An interesting, well-written, accessible publication with excellent recipes.

Meditation for Busy People, Dawn Groves (San Rafael, CA: New World Library, 1992). A practical, easy-to-understand description of how to meditate. Written for the busy businessperson, this book includes useful tips on fitting meditation into a busy schedule and practical advice on meditating in the workplace. Motivating and reassuring.

Videotapes

Yoga Practice for Beginners (Venice, CA: Healing Arts). Produced by the editors of *Yoga Journal*, this videotape is designed for beginners of all fitness levels. It is a high quality, inspiring video. The postures are demonstrated beautifully, with great detail.

Your Healing Breath (Red Hook, NY: Ruella Frank). Ruella Frank demonstrates a variety of deep breathing techniques meant to replenish energy and soothe the mind. She illustrates these techniques in supine and standing positions. Excellent training for beginners.

Energize with Yoga (Cambridge, MA: Rudra Press). Lilias Folan has been teaching yoga on PBS television for years. In this video she demonstrates yoga postures that increase vitality. Excellent for beginners, her explanations are clear, her style is simple, and her enthusiasm is infectious.

Appendix 2

Common Questions

About the Author

DAWN GROVES is a minister, author, and educator. She is also a keynote motivational speaker well-known for her dynamic teaching style, warm presence, and accessible wisdom. Dawn clearly addresses the challenges of people who are attempting to combine professional achievement, spiritual growth, and a balanced lifestyle. She teaches workshops and classes for the government, private industry, community colleges, and spiritual centers throughout the United States and Canada.

For information about Dawn's lectures, workshops, classes, and tapes, please contact Dawn directly at:

HERON HOUSE
P.O. Box 5642
Bellingham, WA 98227
Internet: dawng@nas.com